Well written, informative, clear and very personal. And frankly very *brave*. If I were still treating *psychiatric patients* I'd absolutely advise them to read it. *~Dr. Sturla Bruun-Meyer, Psychiatrist*

Really lets the world know what it's like to LIVE the diagnosis of bipolar disorder. Should be *compulsory reading* for all health professionals. *~Barbara Webster, RN, BScN, MSc.*

Riveting. This book is *for everyone*, including medical personnel, to understand the illness from the patient's point of view. *~Marilyn Ghadirian*

Couldn't put it down. Very well written, and this *compelling* story is at once personal, enlightening, and inspiring. *~Karen Armstrong, Librarian*

If you ever wanted to know what it's like to live through the ups and downs of "bipolar country", this is the book for you! It's a *gripping*, sometimes humorous account... *~Helen Fyles*

Captivating, told with *stunning sincerity*. *~Ryan Kenick*

Hammond is a strong, brave woman. To document her journey into bipolar disorder and share it with others is *remarkable*. *~Elise Titman*

Wow; *bullseye!* The *definitive* book for bipolar sufferers and everyone around them. I was *mesmerized. Read this!* *~Laurence Potgieter*

Amazing! Compelling. Infused with *humour* yet filled with serious research, it permits the reader to enter the incredible labyrinth of the human brain. *A must-read*. *~Anne Vrana*

What a read! The book comes alive. The photos really add to the telling. *A great achievement*. ~*Phyllis Fisher*

Hammond's *courage* and that of the whole family touched me. And the book made me smile so often: that was an unexpected surprise and *delight* given the difficult subject matter. ~*Sandra Norris*

One word: *Wow!* What an *incredible* resource. It allows us to peek right inside the mind of a bipolar sufferer. The appendices are especially helpful. *Indispensable*. ~*Pierre-Julien Mazenot*

I couldn't put it down! This *deeply personal* account takes us into the heart of a life experience that is normally so obscured. Her candor is *riveting*. ~*Helen DeMarsh*

I was sucked right in. It gave me a *deeper understanding* of what my family members with bipolar have dealt with… and how we can *support a loved one* dealing with it. ~*Sue Canfield*

An *insightful* journey into madness and back… A personal account with a researcher's attention to detail and relevant literature… It raises many questions about the indistinct boundary between sanity and madness. ~*Jim Fyles*

Hammond clearly explains how her disorder affected everyone around her. *A must-read*. ~*Alain Brunet, Author of "Good As News"*

A fast and furious read, *riveting* on account of the subject matter, the searing honesty, the wry humour, and the excellent writing. A unique quality is the attention given to the impact of her illness on family dynamics… ~*5-star review posted by Jiminy on Amazon.com*

MAD LIKE ME:

TRAVELS IN BIPOLAR COUNTRY

Mad Like Me

Travels in Bipolar Country

Merryl Hammond, PhD

CAE Canada, 6 Sunny Acres, Baie-D'Urfé, QC, Canada, H9X 3B6

cae.canada@icloud.com

Edited by Tami Hammond-Collins

Second Edition

Disclaimer: This is a memoir – a personal account of the author's own experience with mental illness. Bipolar disorder is an extremely serious disorder, so please always consult your physician or health care provider before using any information or advice in this book. Using ideas from this book is at the sole discretion of the reader. The author and publisher are not liable for any damages resulting from the use of any advice or information in this book. Nevertheless, the author hopes that her story and the self-care strategies she outlines will be helpful to readers on their own "travels in bipolar country."

Archived at the National Library of Quebec

Hammond, Merryl, 1956–

Mad Like Me: Travels in Bipolar Country / Merryl Hammond.

ISBN 978-0-9876788-8-1

Printed in the United States

For video clips, media reports, etc., please see www.merrylhammond.com.

Cover: *Portraits painted by my daughter, Tami Hammond-Collins. On the left, I'm (hypo)manic, and on the right, depressed.*

Dedication

For Rob and all our children. Thank you, thank you for your understanding, acceptance and support.

For all my fellow travellers in Bipolar Country who are "mad like me." With time, patience, consistent treatment, and commitment to self-care, you *can* recover. Take courage. May some of the mistakes I made and lessons I learned guide you on your journey to recovery.

Contents

Foreword

Clinicians have written many academic textbooks about bipolar disorder based on observation and research. This book is not one of them. Rather, it is an elucidating work by a brilliant woman with bipolar disorder who shares her thoughtful personal experiences with this illness.

Bipolar disorder, also known as manic-depressive illness, is characterized by significant shifts of mood, energy and activity. In this well-written and insightful book, Dr. Hammond chronicles her valuable experience with candor, humor and remarkable clarity. She bravely shares some of the darkest moments of her depression and takes us with her as she soars to a state of sublime and powerful excitement in mania.

She eloquently discusses the depth of her suffering when depressed, describing it as "soul-sapping and brain-draining." During the hypomanic or manic phase, however, she was highly elated and admits that she enjoyed every moment! Biological changes in brain activities are responsible for these "wild rides" associated with bipolar disorder.

Her journey into the uncharted and unpredictable territory of bipolar disorder reflects human vulnerability in the face of this serious disease over which one has no effective control. In the initial stages, it might be hard to differentiate between normal excitement and illness. However, family and friends who witness the patient's behaviour soon realize that a significant change is taking place – one that requires intervention by a health professional. Seeking and following a physician's advice is essential to avoid recurrence of the illness.

Hammond's own "Travels in Bipolar Country" were fraught with unexpected surprises, emotional outbursts, and an initial stubborn refusal to accept the reality of her diagnosis. She could not accept that she really had a mental illness. Denial of mental illness is largely related to fear of stigma and public shaming and discrimination. It is unfortunate that in the 21st century and in a country that is so advanced in science and whose citizens are well-educated, many patients who suffer from mental illness still feel that they need to hide or deny a disorder which could be effectively treated. Instead, they become disabled and endure untold suffering. Today in many countries of the world, the stigma – rather than the illness itself – is the most serious obstacle to recovery. Moreover, despite significant progress in the behavioural sciences worldwide, psychiatric patients are still not treated like non-psychiatric ones.

Eventually, as Hammond's mood cycles stabilized with medication and various associated therapies, she began to enjoy better health. What is very touching in her journey is the unceasing accompaniment and support of her family and their tireless sacrifices. This demonstrates a compassion with caring acceptance not often witnessed.

Readers of this book will come to appreciate some of the major challenges of mental illness such as denial and stigma, and the need to respect the dignity of patients and to have compassion and empathy for them.

~ A-M. Ghadirian, M.D.

Professor Emeritus, McGill University, Montreal;
Distinguished Life Fellow of the American Psychiatry Association;
Author of *Creative Dimensions of Suffering*

Thanks

First, I thank my remarkable and uncomplaining husband, Rob Collins. You have been my mainstay during all my wild travels in Bipolar Country, from the scary days before we had a diagnosis but you knew with absolute certainty that I was "off" (while I vehemently denied it), through all the dramas of this mercurial disorder, into and out of the hospital… and finally during the past several years as I have doggedly clawed my way back to health. Rob, despite the ups and downs our relationship has experienced since I got sick, I want you to know that I truly appreciate everything you have done – and are doing – for me on this journey.

"Thank you" doesn't even begin to say it.

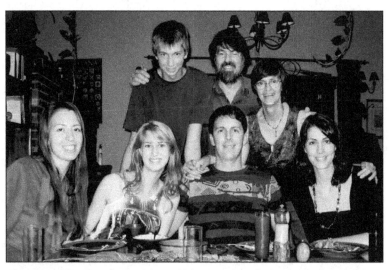

This photo of Rob and me with our kids was taken during a relatively calm moment for me at the start of my bipolar journey in 2008. That's Karrie seated on the left, beside Tami, Kai and Mika; Matt is standing next to Rob, and I'm crouching, as if to form a bridge between the two rows.

Second, I warmly acknowledge our five children, each of whom has experienced at least something of my madness: Kai, living in Botswana; Mika, in Toronto; Karrie, who was here in Montreal for the early crisis phases; Tami, studying, travelling and living at home when I was so ill; and Matt, studying fine arts.

I love you all.

Third, I thank my friends and distant family members who supported me throughout. While some were initially bewildered by the news of mental illness, they tried to stand by me and make me feel better about myself. Thanks to you all. Special thanks to my stepmom, Kristin Hammond, my many siblings (Alan Langbridge, Janet Kennedy, Gillian van der Meulen, Bridget Meiring, Stephen Langbridge, Roan Hammond and Warren Hammond), and to other family and friends – scattered around the world but who felt close when I needed them: Andrew Orkin and Cheryl Levitt, Norman and Sandy Norris, my dear late friend Navid Naimi and her husband Saeed, Leyla Shodjai, Lida Berghuis, Phyllis Fisher, Guicha Barreto, Barbara Webster, Jane Dawson, Judith Quinn, Elizabeth Howard and the rest of the *Mothering Matters* gang, Maury Miloff and Helen deMarsh, Pam Clough, and Gordon Russell.

Fourth, I acknowledge all the helpers and health professionals, both alternative and mainstream, who treated me as both an outpatient and inpatient during the early, rocky stages of the disorder and more recently, since I have "settled." They include acupuncturists, naturopaths, family physicians, psychiatrists, neuropsychologists, psycho-educators, counsellors, nurses, meditation instructors, mindfulness-based cognitive therapy experts, and facilitators at a bipolar therapy group.

I am thinking of Dr. Cheryl Levitt, Mitra Javanmardi, Kim Corbett, Ann St Amant, Judith Quinn, Dr. Sturla Bruun-Meyer, staff at the Herzl Family Practice Centre, Jewish General Hospital, the psychiatrist at that hospital who first diagnosed me and asks to be referred to simply as "Dr. Y" (not his initial), Dr. Eric Lillie, Dr. Suzane Renaud (my psychiatrist at the Douglas Mental Health University Institute), Rebecca Sablé, Dr. Marc-Alain Wolf, the two exceptional nurses who made me feel respected and human as an inpatient, and who I recall only as Nathalie and Robert, Lucy Lu, Joseph Emet, Rosi Di Meglio, Anton Chow and Alla Sernea, Nancy Poirier, Daniel Kunin and Lucia Zaccardelli.

It's a long list, for sure, but it takes many resources to tackle the bipolar beast.[1]

Fifth, I thank all my fellow bipolar sufferers who have published their stories so we can learn from them. (See the list of recommended readings at the end of the book for some of my favourite resources.) We have to work together to end the stigma of this and other mental illnesses. We must remember – and make it clear to others – that we are people with a chronic disease, no more shameful than diabetes, arthritis, or cancer.

Finally, thanks to you, the reader, for considering what I say here and for "being there" in a way that makes me feel connected to a worldwide community of people affected – either directly or indirectly – by bipolar disorder.

---

[1] Staff at the Douglas Mental Health University Institute where I am currently being treated asked me to emphasize to Montreal readers that they do not provide assessment or consultation services by phone or email to people who have not been referred to or are not being followed by a clinical program at the Institute. They advise: "Please consult your doctor or community clinic, or, in case of a mental health emergency, go to an emergency ward or crisis centre."

If you have bipolar disorder and are mad like me, we share not only the diagnosis but no doubt a commitment to recovery. If your loved one has bipolar and is mad like me, thank you for taking the time to inform yourself so you can better understand what s/he may be experiencing in Bipolar Country.

Either way, I hope this book will both inform and inspire you.

Prologue

The idea for this book came at the height of my first full-blown manic episode in 2009. Despite the wild fizzing in my brain, I kept a detailed paper trail of post-it notes with scribbled ideas and insights that enabled me to look back with startling clarity, and to re-live much of what I experienced during those turbulent three weeks. Those notes allowed me to capture realistic recollections of my lurching journey through Bipolar Country.

My goal in this book is not merely to bring you along for the ride, a passive observer of the crazy antics of one particular bipolar sufferer. Rather, I hope to bring you all the way into my stormy mind, so you can experience something of what I went through as a rapid cycling bipolar patient. To achieve this, I need to open the books and practise full disclosure. That won't be easy, but I undertake to try. In return, I ask only that you don't judge me too harshly. And that you take what you learn from my story to inform either your own recovery as a bipolar patient, or your journey supporting a loved one, friend, colleague or client with bipolar. Or both.

Bipolar caused me to disappear from the stage of my own life for two full years, from the age of 51 to 53. I was exiled, lost, shocked, confused and ashamed. If some of the things I share here can help you to shorten your quarantine period in Bipolar Country, I'll be thankful. I've been there. I know how extremely scary and lonely it gets. But I'm here to tell you that things *can* get better, and that you can, piece by piece, build a life where bipolar no longer controls you. You can tame this tiger!

Introduction: First exposures

1976. I'm a 19-year-old student nurse in South Africa, doing a rotation at a sprawling psychiatric hospital that's banished to the outskirts of Pietermaritzburg. We get bused in every morning from the nurses' residence at the general hospital in the city centre. As the bus rattles up to the imposing hospital gates for our first dreaded shift, I peer out, anxious to see for myself the sinister and fearful asylum I had heard so much about from our more senior nursing peers.

It was part of the deal, listening to horror stories from older students about the "mad house," the "loony bin." Everyone had her favourite tales to tell, each more disquieting and distressing than the last. Some of the stories poked fun at the patients and their crazed antics; others at the visitors and even the staff – some of whom we all thought should be patients themselves!

By the end of my rotation, I had my own little stack of anecdotes, filed away and ready to pull out whenever the need arose. There was the patient who had electroconvulsive therapy – which in those days was quite brutal to observe, let alone experience – and became totally amnesiac as a result; the man suffering from toxic psychosis: he had had a bad reaction to street drugs of some kind, and had physically attacked his wife while hallucinating – I was terrified of him, and gave him a wide berth; the drop-dead gorgeous surfer boy who had plummeted into an inexplicable, bottomless depression; the elderly man who had had a lobotomy back in the 1950s when the surgery was popular, who followed us around like a faithful puppy, trying to stroke our hair; the catatonic woman, curled up in a corner, who had been systematically gang-raped by her husband's friends every weekend while he looked on. ("Who's the mad one in that relationship?" we whispered, appalled.) And then there were the ungodly howls and shrieks from the isolation ward we students were never allowed to enter.

Punctuating our almost uniformly ineffective attempts to relate to our patients, there were awkward interactions with jaded staff members who scoffed at any small humane gestures we made towards our patients, any pitiful efforts to treat them as human beings rather than caged lunatics. And there were the gaunt visitors, fearful, furtive, ashamed to be there because their mere presence announced to the world that a loved one was tainted by madness.

My treasury of war stories proved that I had been there, done that; earned my stripes. I had been initiated into the ranks of those who had looked mental illness and its − in those days − somewhat barbaric treatment in the eye. I had seen something of the suffering it caused, and what I saw had made me shudder.

Even though much of the physical distress we dealt with in the general hospital was awful in its own way, nothing ever compared with the psychic anguish I had witnessed in the psychiatric hospital. The hopelessness. The blank-eyed vacancy. The impenetrable depression. The loss of autonomy and identity. I was so glad it was over: out of sight, out of mind.

But eight years later, as part of my post-graduate training in community health nursing, I had to do another rotation at a psychiatric hospital in Johannesburg, South Africa's largest city. Older and hopefully more compassionate by then, and with the benefit of my limited previous experience in Pietermaritzburg, I felt a bit less apprehensive at the start.

That didn't last long.

The first thing I heard when I entered the ward was distraught wailing that got louder and more unnerving with each breath. This young mother had given birth a month earlier and plunged into a paralyzing postpartum depression soon after. Now she was here, howling like a banshee, evidently re-living some anguished experience over and over again, and submitting all the other patients – and the poor staff – to her screeching, while her newborn was off in foster care. When I bravely tried to approach her, to talk to her, distract her with my kindness, she reacted violently, screaming even louder and kicking out at me. Well, that went well! I looked over my shoulder and saw two of the permanent staff snickering at my naiveté.

There was a young man I privately referred to as "Torch" who had miraculously survived massive third degree burns after dousing himself with gas and setting himself alight before sprinting, screaming, around the yard "to punish his parents" for making his life so miserable. I would not have liked to be their family therapist, I thought.

There was a skeletal young woman with life-threatening anorexia, a nasogastric tube taped to her nose so she could be force-fed. I had no idea how to comfort her: she seemed to hate herself so much that she just wanted to melt away and die.

There was a middle-aged man whose entire life had been derailed by obsessive-compulsive disorder: he was compelled to wash his hands after touching anything – a door-knob, plate, fork, magazine, counter, pill, whatever. Just imagine. I tried valiantly to engage and distract him, but he constantly rushed off to wash in mid-sentence.

And there was a woman with mania: talking so loudly and so fast I couldn't understand her most of the time; she'd laugh hysterically at any slight provocation, and refuse to sit down to eat, she was so elated and "speeded up." I had never seen anything like this and was frankly baffled by her.

During this rotation, I was aware of feeling uncomfortably hypocritical. As a nurse, I knew it was my job – my duty – to care for these patients, regardless of the mental state they were in. If they had been patients in a general hospital – vomiting, bleeding, incontinent, pus draining from open wounds, cancerous growths protruding from rotting flesh, whatever – I wouldn't have thought twice about cleaning them up, making them comfortable, setting them at ease. But here, in a mental hospital, faced with the psychic equivalents of those physical signs of illness, my patients' behaviours mystified and often repelled me. At some deep level, I feared them. I judged them. I blamed them. I stigmatized them.

"Why doesn't she just snap out of it?" "Get a grip!" "Control yourself, woman!" "Just grow up and stop seeking attention." "He's just avoiding responsibility." And so on.

I did not see them as full human beings.

And secretly, I felt superior to them. I had it all together, while they were just a total mess.

Admitting that now sickens me. After all, I had taken the Nightingale Pledge, part of which states: "May my life be devoted to service and to the high ideals of the nursing profession."

Each morning of that second rotation, I drove through the hospital gates with the best intentions, and at the end of each shift I fled, defeated and disheartened. There was so little I could do to bring relief to any of these patients. It was as if they were from another planet: I didn't understand their language, their customs, their needs.

How could I be "devoted to service" under these impossible conditions?

I was so grateful when the rotation was finally over, and grateful, too, that I was mentally well. That I'd never again have to walk through the locked doors of a psychiatric ward.

Ha! Famous last words.

Part 1:

Build-up to bipolar

Chapter 1: Before bipolar

I had a rather non-exceptional childhood. Looking back, there were no telling signs, no show-stoppers, no a-ha moments that I could point to and say: "There! *That's* what triggered me to be susceptible to bipolar disorder!"

I was born in 1956 in Johannesburg, South Africa. My parents divorced when I was seven, and both eventually remarried. As a result, I was lucky enough to have two loving parents, two equally loving stepparents, a biological sister, two stepsisters, two stepbrothers, and two half-brothers. This was the sizable brood with which I grew up, perfectly contentedly for the most part.

Schooling was largely uneventful, with my final two years spent at a boarding school in Potchefstroom, which – despite my initial trepidation – I really loved.

I studied at the University of Natal in Durban, and graduated as a nurse and midwife in 1978. At age eighteen, during my second year in university, I fell in love. We dated for seven long years before finally getting married (after much arm-twisting from me) in Johannesburg in 1982. After such a long courtship, I was sure we'd be safe. No such luck. Two years later, we divorced (my decision).

While still in that relationship, I did first an Honours and then a Master's degree in Sociology.

In 1984, freshly divorced, I started living with my colleague and new love, Rob Collins, in Gazankulu, a remote homeland established by the apartheid government where we were both working on a progressive rural primary health care program. During this time, I was accepted as a PhD candidate in adult education and community health at the University of the Witwatersrand in Johannesburg. I got my doctorate in 1989.

With Rob came – part-time at least – my two beautiful stepchildren, Kai, then aged six, and Mika, four. Thanks to them pressuring us, we married in 1987. My first biological child, Karrie, was born in Johannesburg in 1988.

When Karrie was only four months old, we emigrated from South Africa to Canada, settling in suburban Montreal. We left because we had been active in the anti-apartheid movement, and felt the threat of impending military service for Rob. Fortunately, we were able to leave without becoming exiles, so were free to return to visit Kai and Mika – who then lived with their mom in Cape Town – and the rest of our family members.

I tried to adjust to Canada with gusto. Maybe too much gusto. Our second winter here, I decided to show all our hibernating neighbours how to do it. One sunny January morning, I strapped Karrie into her baby seat on the back of my bike and went cycling gleefully down the street. The roads had been cleared of snow, so I felt perfectly safe. Only later, in agony in hospital, awaiting surgery on my thoroughly fractured femur, I reflected on the difference between "snow-cleared" and "safe" streets. I now have an extremely healthy respect for black ice. And I humbly respect the annual hibernation period that most wise Canadians choose to observe…

My second child, Tami, was born in 1991 in Montreal; and finally, Matt in 1992.

For the first several years in Canada, I was busy taking care of our young children, and was an active volunteer for

environmental and social justice causes. During this time, I
started two grassroots organizations, both of which I headed
up for about ten years. The first was *Mothering Matters,* a support group for at-home mothers which eventually had many
chapters in the Montreal-area and beyond. We got federal
funding for some of our projects to raise the profile of women
who choose to stay home to raise their children. The second
was *Citizens for Alternatives to Pesticides,* which called for a mor-
atorium on the cosmetic use of pesticides in residential areas
until their safety had been proven. We lobbied for and got
local bylaws banning pesticide use in many towns, recruited
spokespeople from across Canada, met with many government officials including the federal Minister of Health, and
did countless media reports. I also served as chair of the local
Baie-D'Urfé Citizens' Association during this time.

In 1994, I joined the Baha'i Faith, and true to form,
jumped in and volunteered to teach children's classes, serve
on an Education Committee, write and edit educational resources, and so on. I had always been a high achiever, perfectionist, workaholic. Rob, who had for many years been
advising me to "slow down" and "just say no" to various volunteer commitments, just shook his head in disbelief: yet another cause to swallow my energy and keep me busy-busy...

So why not add yet another source of stress to the mix?
I had not worked for pay since Karrie was born. I missed my
career. With Matt, Tami and Karrie being two, four and
seven years old, I felt ready to start taking on some part-time
consulting work. Staff at the Jewish General Hospital and
McGill University in Montreal needed someone with my
skills to work on a tobacco control project. It was perfect for
me: academic research, summarizing data, writing up results
in a user-friendly way, consulting with a team of like-minded

educators – all things I loved to do. This work resulted in two publications, both targeting family physicians.

That first break into the Canadian job market soon led to other offers, and tobacco control – especially in Inuit and First Nations communities – became a major area of interest for over twenty years, till today. This work has resulted in the publication of many books, reports, articles and conference papers, and the production of several educational videos.

I tell you all this only to show that I was a capable and productive worker, initiating and sustaining projects, managing my own time, and balancing family responsibilities, paid work, travel in the Far North and numerous volunteer commitments.

Then one day early in 2008, the phone rang. When the caller identified herself and explained the reason for the call, my chest constricted and I gasped for air. This was going to have monumental significance in my life. It started the chain of events that eventually led to me driving myself mad.

Bipolar was looming.

Chapter 2: Playing with fire

The phone call and ensuing crisis involved one of our kids at school. (Please bear with me as I withhold specific details of this incident, to protect the child concerned.) I was hugely emotionally invested in saving the situation and protecting not only our child, but our entire family's reputation. So there was a major "mother bear" factor, on top of the physical and emotional burnout caused by frantically fighting the system: educational authorities at all levels up to and including the Minister of Education, and law enforcement officials.

This became my latest cause. Overwrought, I worked eighteen-hour days, seven days a week, with occasional all-nighters while preparing for big meetings to defend our child. It went on for five fraught weeks. I made no time to eat, so Rob brought finger-food to the desk in my home office. (He and I run a public health consultancy and work from home when we are not travelling to work with our colleagues in Inuit and First Nations communities.) Dishes piled up in the sink, and the laundry room looked like there was a fire sale going on in there. I filled two thick ring binders with notes, printouts and documents.

I was intensely fired up and had emotional tunnel vision; reason and objectivity were totally eclipsed.

There was one incident when I was on the phone to an authority figure on one line, and Rob strode in with the cordless phone saying that another key person was returning my call on the other line. I needed to ask them both the same question, so I had my phone pressed to one ear, the cordless phone to the other, and I was barking at both people simultaneously, flipping pages in my ring binder with my elbows!

Even I should have realized there was something wrong with this picture.

Long hours were nothing new to me: I had worked hard many, many times before, meeting project deadlines, completing theses, publishing textbooks, and so on. But the extent of the hours and the duration of this crisis were new. As well, this time, two critical elements were different.

First, there was the desperate emotional investment: this involved one of our precious children who – in our opinion – was being maligned by powerful and unfeeling authority figures and therefore needed our wholehearted protection.

Second, menopause. I was 51 at the time and had recently started full-blown menopausal symptoms. I have often wondered what role menopause – with her volatile hormones – played in triggering my mental illness, or in making it worse than it otherwise would have been.

I wonder which of these factors had a greater influence on my extreme reaction to this family crisis? No way to know.

Either way, I did absolutely everything I could to resolve matters, with no success.

Looking back, I should never have tried to fight the perceived injustice. I should have let it go, accepted the situation and moved on without outrage or obsession. I should have taken up kick-boxing instead! Had I done that, I truly believe I would not be here, now, writing about my experiences with bipolar disorder.

By choosing the path of greatest resistance, I literally drove myself mad.

Chapter 3: Depression descends

"People who haven't experienced actual depression can't imagine how debilitating it is. I felt hopeless, helpless." ~Friedlander (2010:163)

"I couldn't get out of bed. I had no self-esteem and felt beaten down by life." ~Avrutis (2010:66)

First depression

My frenzied exertions to get justice for our child were, in hindsight, part of my first hypomanic episode. (Please see Appendix 1 for definitions.) It was followed by a severe depression.

On May 19, 2008, I finally accepted defeat concerning the family crisis, and told everyone that I couldn't keep going any longer. Did I weep? I don't remember, but if I didn't weep on the outside, I sure did on the inside. I felt that despite my most inspired and spirited efforts, I had utterly failed as a mother.

Nevertheless, I knew it was time to tidy my desk, filing away the piles of notes that had accumulated during the crisis and shelving the heavy – both literally and figuratively – ring binders from the drama. I started to shuffle the mounds of work-related papers and mail that had lain neglected all those weeks, but nothing looked at all appealing. I checked my overflowing email inbox, but it all felt way too overwhelming.

No problem, I thought, we'll take this slowly. First thing is to rest a bit. I surely deserved that!

But rest was not the answer.

Depression descended within four days of my admitting defeat. I became listless and moody. I dreaded a social event planned at our home and told Karrie and Rob that they were on their own hosting it. I had zero energy. When my friend, Navid, saw me at the event, she immediately expressed concern about how drained I looked, and was the first one to say the dreaded D-word to me: "Maybe you're depressed?"

Don't be silly, I snapped. I don't get depressed! I guess I'm just a bit tired…

"I don't get depressed." Yeah, right.

Within a day or two of what turned out to be her perfectly correct diagnosis, I had all the classic signs and symptoms of full-blown depression. It descended as resolutely as an automatic garage door rumbling closed. I was trapped inside, in the dank, dark, tomb-like garage, knowing the sun was beaming just beyond the door that I was utterly powerless to open.

If you've never experienced depression, let me try to describe how it felt.

Dulled senses

All my senses were dampened and muted. My eyes felt unfocused. Colours were paler, muddied with grey. Sounds were muffled: everything seemed to be coming through a soundproofed wall – it was hard to hear and took too much energy to decipher. My taste buds were withered: food was insipid and unappetizing. My sense of touch was deadened: I had no interest in intimacy or human contact with anyone.

The whole world was enveloped in a sick, thick fog, toxic to all who were exposed.

Physical symptoms

I was physically exhausted in depression. It was not just bone-deep, it was marrow-deep. Nothing I did could shake it. My limbs felt like lead, and just the thought of moving made me tired.

I was overwhelmed by the smallest physical tasks. Taking out the garbage dismayed me. One night, after finally doing so, weakly staggering back from the curb, I looked up at the sky and saw the stars. "My God, it's all too much for me." I crawled upstairs to my trusty bed and collapsed like a rag doll, spent.

Urinating took at least five or ten minutes. I would sit and stare at the wall in front of me, and zone out completely. I'd hear Rob's voice on the phone in his home office, murmuring endlessly through the wall. I was deep underwater, flailing and sinking while he swam confidently and carelessly above me. Just the effort of getting up from a seated position was too strenuous: I'll just sit here for a while longer.

The only moments of pleasure I had during the day were when I prowled off and collapsed either on the bed or the couch and drifted off into a stress-relieving nap. The escape I experienced then was truly lifesaving – I could not have managed without these oases in the depression desert.

Sleep was my only solace, offering brief oblivion. More than that: sleep was a clandestine lover from whom I couldn't bear to be separated. I wanted only to be wrapped in his protective arms, and have the world eclipsed by his tender attentions. Wakefulness was the ultimate enemy. With wakefulness came people. Responsibilities. Commitments. Guilt. Energy-draining chores. Forget it; just roll over and try to blot it all out.

But this lover, sleep, was not at all welcome in our home. His unwanted presence during the day meant that I was deep in a hole. So I had to sneak around to make time for my liaisons with him. Every time I snuck off to lie down, I was filled with self-loathing. You're hopeless, I thought. But I was too weighed down by exhaustion to get up. Hour after hour passed like this. I made earnest promises to myself: I'll definitely get up at 3 p.m. But 3 p.m. came and went. I pretended not to notice the time, or I bargained with myself. Okay, 4 p.m. No such luck. I swear, at 4:30 I'll get up. Finally, Rob would come up to see how I was doing at about 5:30, and I'd tell him I'd come down later for dinner. (He or one of the children was cooking for us. I had long ago forsaken that role.)

I dreaded meals with a vengeance. At dinnertime I finally crept downstairs, feeling sick that I had let yet another afternoon pass on the bed, and even sicker at the thought of having to eat actual food: my stomach was as deeply depressed as my brain was. It wasn't just that I had no appetite; food actually turned my stomach. As well, the whole family was there, each person stealthily assessing my progress – or lack thereof. Could I allay their anxieties if I forced a few mouthfuls of this abominable stuff down my tightly clenched throat into my anxiously knotted stomach? Could I fool them that I was feeling a bit better, at last? Or would my dark-ringed eyes, hollowed out cheeks, down-turned mouth and slumped shoulders give away my true state? Bravely, I tried to straighten my back and compose my face for the children and Rob: what must it be like to watch your mother/wife literally fade away like this? Lord knows, I didn't want *them* to feel depressed on my account.

Finally, it would officially be time for bed. Another dreadful day done. At least now I could go to bed like a "normal" person, without guilt. Needless to say, our bed served only to cradle my tormented body and mind. There was no sex whatsoever. It would have been like Rob making love to a corpse, that's how much energy and desire I had in that state. Rob instinctively kept his distance, respecting my anguish.

But then, night after night, sleep cruelly eluded me. I'd lie stiffly, trying not to disturb Rob who was exhausted from the stress of my illness, while maddeningly repetitive, circular thoughts and fears tormented my fuzzy brain.

Emotional numbing

Emotionally, I was sidelined. I felt completely melancholic and hollow. Those whom I loved most in the world shrank in significance. Not only were they smaller than before but they were separated from me by a thick glass barrier that imprisoned me in a helpless emotional vacuum. I knew intellectually how a "good wife and mother" should behave, but there was no way I could reach out to them. I wanted nothing to do with them emotionally. I was an icy bitch.

I felt so joyless I forgot how to smile. Laughter was an empty echo from some former age. Things that normally pleased or thrilled me meant nothing now. I couldn't imagine what all the fuss had been about before. For example, if one of the children did well at school, or the dog did something cute, or the gulls were crying out overhead, or the girls were baking cookies from scratch... Normally, these things would have delighted me. Now, I could not care less. There was darkness and no consolation. I felt utterly cheerless. No *joie de vivre*.

For a college project, Tami painted a blue portrait of me in depression, with sunken eyes, a miserable, thin face and a turned-down mouth (see below and front cover). When I look at it now, I remember all those times when I felt so joyless I forgot how to smile; when laughter was an empty echo.

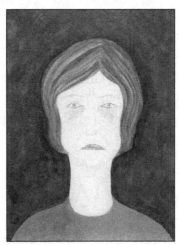

Tami's "depression portrait" of me.

Intellectual apathy

Perhaps scariest of all, the intellectual part of my brain switched off. The neurons were disconnected; the battery was flat. I felt thick-headed; my mind was leaden. Thoughts couldn't travel through it at normal speed, and emotions were dragged down to the depths and got mired there. I was an intellectual zombie.

When I went back over my agendas preparing to write this book, it was so clear how my lack of physical and intellectual energy played out in day-to-day life. Weeks and weeks went by where there was nothing at all written in my agenda. Then gradually, as I recovered, a sprinkling and then a normal amount of appointments reappeared.

Working was out of the question. It took way too much energy and focus. For someone who had always been a shameless workaholic, this inability to work was incomprehensible.

Rob gently suggested that I try doing a bit of work with him in his office. I would sit there, trying to listen to him talk to our colleagues on a conference call. He used speakerphone so I could join in whenever I liked.

I didn't like.

I had nothing useful to say. My mouth was drained of words. They had fled and were stowed deep in the rumpled recesses of my troubled brain. I would look away from the desk, trying to find anything in the office to interest me. Nothing. Dear God, I was so disconnected. So out of it. I just wanted to lie down. I forced myself to sit a while longer. By now, my mind had gone totally blank: I didn't even know the topic of the call any more. Rob's voice droned on. What language was he speaking, I wondered? It might as well have been Latin! I knew I should be able to say something, to respond intelligently, but I simply could not. Before long, I got so restless and frustrated, I'd signal to Rob that I had to leave and stagger out. He'd nod understandingly, and later, come upstairs to find me curled on the bed, my back to the door, hating myself for letting him down yet again.

If I'd had any tears in me, I would have wept dejectedly.

My home office is just at the foot of the stairs, so every time I came down from the bedroom to the main floor, I saw my neglected desk with unopened mail and other papers piling up, clamouring for attention. Bookshelves brimmed with evidence of a long and productive career: thick ring binders filled with notes and outputs from every project I have worked on in Canada – over sixty of them; my computer bulging with digital folders and files; my fax machine, scanner and printer – all lying dormant, anxious to be pressed into service again. The forsaken office filled me with shame and guilt. I couldn't stand the pressure.

I clicked the door closed and walked past, ignoring the backlog.

What else could I do? I was like some ancient mechanical merry-go-round, broken down, with no parts to repair it. So much intellectual potential, all wasted, all lost now.

Social isolation

I felt almost totally disconnected from my family and friends. I became acutely self-centred, consumed with my own inner turmoil. I expected everyone to realize how engulfed I was, and to make appropriate allowances for me. As the weeks passed, I felt a rift widening between all my family members and myself.

As I said, I'd often creep off to nap during the day. I preferred going upstairs to my bed, where I'd normally be left in peace. Collapsing on the couch was comforting in a pinch, but there I always risked having people loitering around me, trying to cheer me up or make light conversation. But I was beyond cheer, and no conversation was light; it was all heavy, requiring focus, responses, strength I didn't have.

As for my friends, I didn't have energy to stay in touch or pretend that I was socially competent, so I simply withdrew.

Like any wounded animal would.

I didn't want to see anyone when I was in this state. Two of my best friends would sometimes pop by unannounced while out on a walk together, to invite me to join them, or just to stay and chat for a while, clearly trying to cheer me up, to bring me glad tidings. Well, guess what. All tidings were sad. "Just leave me alone," I wanted to yell. If I'd had the stamina to yell.

I was a lump of inertia: careless, friendless, soulless.

Suicidal thoughts

I was lost in thick woods with no paths and didn't know which way to turn to get back to me.

I was caught in quicksand; depression sucked me down, suffocating me.

That first depression lasted six ghastly weeks, until the end of June, and every day I thought I was going to die, I felt so bad. And yes, thoughts of suicide were a constant feature in my muddled, morose mind. To be dead, obliterated, was the finest thing I could imagine.

Depression was soul-sapping, brain-draining. It sucked me down into a dark vortex from which escape felt impossible. Limp-limbed and hollow-eyed, I staggered through the day, longing for escape. I craved the ultimate annihilation.

Maddeningly often, I would lie there waiting for the release of sleep, only to have endlessly circular thoughts plague me. I would stare, doe-eyed, at the ceiling, longing for relief

from the thoughts, fears, ruminations, ceaseless thinking-wor-
rying-fussing. These anxious, repetitive, blacker-than-black
ideas almost inevitably left me lying stiffly on my back, imagining I was in my grave. I could feel the hard, cold coffin beneath me, and I saw only blackness around me. It wasn't scary
at all; rather, strangely comforting. At last, oblivion. Nothing-
ness. Peace.

But then, soon enough, the phone would ring, or Rob
would grind his coffee beans, or the doorbell would chime,
and I'd snap back to reality: no freedom, no void, no grave.
Oh no; I can't stand this.

Looking for treatment

At first, despite all these symptoms, I was in total denial. This
was the first depression I had ever experienced. I didn't even
know what to call it, the feelings were so foreign to me. But
eventually I admitted that something was wrong and chose to
try acupuncture. (Even though I'm a trained nurse, I have
always been open to alternative therapies like naturopathy
and acupuncture.) I had three appointments during the acute
depression phase, and nine more later. It was no miracle cure,
but after the third session I thought I noticed a slight lightening of mood. Whether this was due to the treatments or
simply a factor of the not-yet-diagnosed bipolar disorder is
anyone's guess.

At the end of June, I consulted a psychologist, hoping
for some tips about how to manage this still-unnamed condition. I had dragged myself to her office, feeling wooden, and
resented the cost of an hour with her. Five minutes into the
session, she started asking me inane questions about my child-

hood, how I felt about my mother, and so on. I became exasperated. I hadn't come for an amateurish Freudian analysis, but for concrete information about how I could effectively improve my mood.

I never went back.

I searched online for other psychologists but was put off by the price. I did try one other therapist who came highly recommended by a friend, but never hit it off with her, so only consulted her once.

Rob, in desperation, called the Herzl Family Practice Centre at the Jewish General Hospital to ask for an urgent appointment for assessment. I felt like death so Rob had to drive me. The resident, hearing about my reaction to the family crisis that seemed to have triggered this depression, diagnosed "situational depression," and suggested a wait-and-see approach to treatment, although I was desperate enough to have begged her for anti-depressants – very much against my normal anti-pharmaceutical inclinations. That was the first time, apart from when Navid said it, that I heard the word "depression" attached to me. I felt relieved to hear that she thought the depression was only "situational": that meant it would soon go away as I adjusted to the circumstances that had caused me to get depressed, no?

No.

As it later became clear, this wasn't situational at all. It was, in fact, a depressive episode of undiagnosed bipolar disorder, but it took a second hypomanic episode (the first, during the family crisis, had gone undetected by us all) to leave enough clues for health professionals to make a correct diagnosis.

The photo below was taken in the depths of this desperation when our daughters Karrie and Tami tried to cheer me up by giving me a facial and back massage. They had me trussed up in a shower cap to keep my hair back, and I forced a weak smile, posing self-consciously for the camera. My face was sallow and gaunt from lack of food, my eye sockets shadowed and sunken from anxiety and lack of sleep. I remember that evening of pampering with the girls as one of the few bright spots during the entire ordeal: they still love me!

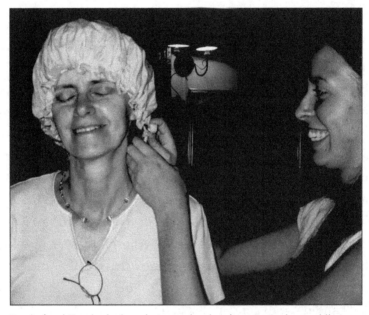

Karrie (and Tami, playing photographer here) pampered me while I was incapacitated by depression.

During the whole of June, Karrie took me under her wide wing and forced me to do daily exercises with her in the basement. I dreaded the exertion, but she was adamant and quite right: it made me feel better, slowly-slowly.

Later, Tami and then Rob took over as my faithful exercise buddies.

Emerging from the depths

When I finally emerged from depression, it was like coming back from the dead; a true resurrection. I had two glorious weeks of normalcy in early July 2008.

I was so happy to be back! After weeks of not having any energy to respond to emails from concerned family members, I wrote to all my family in South Africa:

July 10, 2008.

I'm back!

Just a quick note to tell you that "I'm back!" Completely out of the hole/depression I had fallen into for so many weeks… I'm eating, sleeping, working, and being active again – almost as good as new. What a relief! It feels so GOOD to have my energy back again. Rob was truly amazing through the whole drama – what a good companion he is when times get tough! I really owe him. Thanks to all of you for your kind wishes and concern throughout. Even though you're all far away, it really helped.

Kai arrives from Botswana next Thursday, and Mika will come from Toronto so we'll have all 5 kids here together for a few days. Can't wait! Then Karrie goes to the States for two weeks, and the rest of us will drive to Toronto to see Mika's new condo, and maybe to visit Niagara Falls, etc. Looking forward to a break!

Ah, if only I'd known then about my looming diagnosis and the relentless teeter-totter one is forced to ride in the early stages of this disorder, I would have titled that email "I'm back – for now, but will soon be flying way too high!"

For about two weeks after that first depression, I was stable, like a river happily meandering along at a normal pace. In depression, that river freezes over: it can't move or flow; it's paralyzed. Then, in hypomania, the river hits many rocks, and turns to white-water rapids. Finally, in mania, the river becomes a wild waterfall, racing, plunging and crashing unpredictably over the precipice.

My depression was finally over.

Time for hypomania…

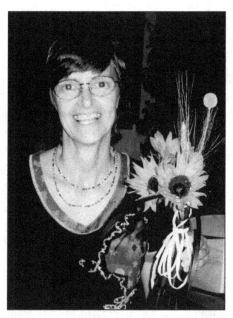

Holding happy sunflowers to welcome Kai from Botswana. Delighted to be "back" from my first depression, July 2008. My smile speaks volumes.

Part 2:

Battling bipolar

Chapter 4: Diagnosis

My journey with bipolar had begun with a workaholic high (meaning: "an unrecognized, undiagnosed hypomanic episode") during our family crisis. At the time, it just looked like "Merryl's working like a demon again, only more so than usual because this involves the good name of her child – and the whole family."

So, what happened as I emerged from that first depression was in fact my second hypomanic episode. Only we didn't yet have words for it, so no expectations, no cautions about how to react to or treat it. We were all flying blind. And was I ever flying! Within two weeks of coming "back" from depression, I careened onto a bumpy high road and left my family way behind in the dust.

When I was in this hypomanic state, having something on or over my head – a hat, a scarf, even a canvas shopping bag! – soothed me. As if it might "contain" or restrain my racing brain.

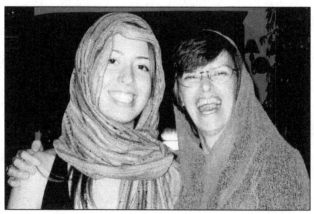

Karrie humoured me and posed with a scarf around her head to match me.

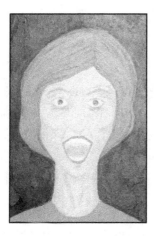

Tami painted this manic-face portrait of me (see front cover) based on the photo above.

This hypomania – which I must admit I thoroughly enjoyed – lasted four glorious weeks. The view from up there was sublime.

I never wanted to descend.

I think this was my "best" episode, in that it wasn't yet full-blown mania – which would require me to physically isolate myself from Rob and the family or be hospitalized – and yet I felt perpetually high, as if I were on some mind-altering substance with no side effects.

I loved every minute of it.

My family hated it.

In the middle of it all, we had scheduled a trip to Toronto and Niagara Falls. We were going to have a full minivan: Rob and me, Kai, Mika, Tami and Matt. (Karrie was away in the United States.)

Everyone was dreading my endless ebullience and constant high-speed chatter. "Oh, wow! Look over there! What a beautiful [you fill in the blank – almost everything looked magnificent to me in that state]!"

"iPoddy"

Someone had the brilliant idea to buy me an iPod to shut me up on the trip. I still remember unwrapping the precious little device: it was tiny, shiny and purple – my favourite colour. The matching purple earbuds made me yelp with delight, they were so diminutive and delicate. One of the children put all my favourite music onto "iPoddy", as I christened her. In no time, I was submerging myself for prolonged periods in the calming waters of songs and music, leaving the family in peace.

That iPod became my best, best friend through this period of hypomania. When I put those earbuds in and closed my eyes to get lost in a song, I literally entered another world, free of the disapproving frowns of my family, their knowing and critical glances at each other, and any lingering doubts I might have had about my state of mind: was there really something wrong with me, after all? My iPod was a first-rate solution to an intractable problem, and it brought much-needed relief to the family and tranquility to me. I highly recommend it!

Tami reflected later that plugging me in to iPoddy was like giving a pacifier to a screaming baby: instant peace and quiet for the rest of the family!

Still having the agonies of depression fresh in my mind, I spent long hours listening closely to the lyrics of sad songs, trying to find kindred spirits who knew what depression (not mere sadness after the loss of a love affair, for example) felt like. I thought that I "diagnosed" quite a few singer-songwriters who had been there, done that, like I had.

Irritability

Just before we were due to leave on the Toronto trip, I experienced my first real flare-up of irrational irritability – a common symptom of (hypo)mania. I don't recall the details, as I
was too buzzy, but I do recall all the family gathered around
the dining room table, looking grave, and me being called in
to be "spoken to." As I entered, I felt exactly like a naughty
schoolgirl summoned to the principal's office. I did not at all
appreciate being patronized by my own children. I soon
huffed and stormed out dramatically.

Mika, braver than the rest, thought things might go better if she spoke to me one-on-one. She asked me to go with
her into the park across from our house, and there, in the
middle of the meadow, tried gently to talk some sense into
me. About what, I don't recall. All I remember is becoming
uncontrollably, blindly enraged with her. I yelled (most uncharacteristic of me, regardless of the provocation, and totally
unthinkable in public) and started to stomp back to the house.
She stepped into my path to block me, still trying to get my
attention, appeal to my rationality, and make her point. I
couldn't believe it! What nerve! Who did she think she was,
treating me with such disrespect? I reached out to push her
away from me, and fortunately she relented before I became
further incited and maybe even violent. I have no doubt that
this altercation might have degenerated if she had stood her
ground any longer.

I don't remember this, but Rob tells me that right after
this scene with Mika, I stormed into the house and angrily
accused Kai, Matt and him (all the guys in the family) of gang-
ing up on me. They were all totally dumbfounded. Rob says
he reassured Kai and Matt: "Don't worry; it'll soon blow
over."

So much conflict. Such drama. I was a heartless hurricane, lashing, thrashing at everything I contacted, showing no mercy. My brain had fierce bolts of lightning emanating from it. Any one of them could have been deadly; the whole storm was unspeakable.

What a great way for us all to start a six-hour journey in a confined space. Time to simmer down with iPoddy's soothing, non-judgmental care.

Off we went. My blood pressure slowly dropped, my red face returned to normal, and my irritability faded until I couldn't even remember what had set me off. I didn't care in the least. That malicious little mental spike had dissipated, and it was as if it had never gripped me. Or so it seemed to me, at least. What scars I had left on the family and on Mika in particular, I did not know. And frankly, I didn't much care. In that state, it was all about *moi*. The rest of them could all just go to hell, as far as I was concerned.

Years later, working on this book, I asked Mika if she remembered that nasty incident in the park. Absolutely! When I read this section to her, she graciously assured me: "Don't worry; I'm scar-free!" At least now, looking back, we know that I was ill – undiagnosed and untreated – at the time, and not responsible for either my vicious and volatile emotions or my erratic and unpredictable actions.

Toronto

After a few minor incidents and a lot of uncharacteristic bickering between Rob and me during the drive, we got to Toronto. We dropped Mika at her home with Kai, who was going to crash on her couch for a few days. They had to get their bags out of the back of the van, so I scrambled out and went around to open the trunk. Rob called out to me to be careful because the van was tightly packed with luggage. He specifically warned that Kai's laptop was on top of everything and could easily slide out. I didn't pay him any attention; I was sick of his endless cautions and lectures. I was in my own world, just doing my own thing. I yanked open the rear door carelessly. Sure enough, Kai's laptop came flying down onto the street. Thank goodness it was in a protective case. Rob vaulted out of the car and rushed to assess the damage, yelling: "I *told* you not to open the door yet. You've broken his laptop, now." Kai, still stuck helplessly in the back seat, was stretched over, arm fully extended out of the trunk, frozen, as if to grab his laptop before it broke free. He was understandably exasperated that it had fallen; Rob was enraged.

I felt humiliated about the laptop, but it was an honest mistake, an accident. I was just trying to be helpful! I didn't deserve to be shouted at. In fact, I took one look at Rob with his florid face and flashing eyes, and simply removed myself from the unseemly scene. I stalked off into Mika's condo building and hid in a quiet corner of the lobby. Eventually, when Rob's rage had subsided, Mika came and found me and I, having cooled off, agreed to join the family again.

Despite the long drive from Montreal and all the emotional dramas – or perhaps because of them – I couldn't sleep. I thrashed and writhed in our hotel bed all night, finally clocking a total of fewer than three hours' sleep.

Even I knew this was neither healthy nor normal.

Yet I felt fine; wide-awake and ripe for adventure. I crept out of the room before 6 a.m. and went to the outdoor pool where I could stride around freely without disturbing Rob. The only soul available for me to chatter with was the young man cleaning the pool. He said he had recently arrived in Canada from China, which I found unimaginably interesting. We talked animatedly for over an hour while he studiously worked, at which time a young woman came to swim. She had not even put down her towel before I called over to introduce the pool cleaner and myself. She, somewhat bemused by all this crack-of-dawn joviality, said she was Jane Parker (not her real name), originally from England but now living in Beijing, visiting Toronto for a business meeting. Beijing! I cannot describe to you the sense of utter awe I felt: two people from China on the pool deck at the same time! It seemed truly miraculous to me. I could not get over it and felt there must be some special significance to it.

Jane finished her laps, and – on a whim – I invited her to breakfast with me. (Forget the family! Jane seemed like much more exciting company to me.) We had a lovely meal together, and I heard all about her travels, work and the project that had brought her to Toronto. I thoroughly enjoyed this break from concerned-looking family members and felt quite normal while I was with her. I then took an arbitrary decision and invited her to join us on our planned trip to Niagara Falls the following day. She was delighted to accept.

That same day, we met up with Kai, Mika, and her boyfriend for a day of sightseeing. I remember three incidents.

First, we walked down to the waterfront, and the plan was that we'd all catch a ferry over to the Toronto Islands to walk along the beach and swim. But on our way to the ferry, we passed a majestic tall ship docked, getting ready to sail on a tour of the harbour. An irrational, overwhelming urge to be on that ship seized me. You could not have spoken any sense into me. I simply had to go! No one else was as enthusiastic as I was, and they actively tried to dissuade me. The more they argued, the more determined I became. "I'm going. You do whatever you want!" And so our big family outing split into two groups, with only Rob (my caretaker, I suppose) and Tami (the peacemaker to ensure that Rob and I didn't fight) accompanying me on by far the most thrilling ride of my life. (None of the other tourists on board seemed quite as enthralled as I was, but then, none of them was in an altered state of consciousness.) That trip was pure at-one-with-nature, wind-in-your-hair joy.

One of the passengers was an elegant woman with grey hair that was cut super-stylishly. I was utterly captivated and thought that style would look great on me. So I made Tami stalk her to get surreptitious photos from all angles, so I could show my hairdresser. Of course, this project of mine deeply embarrassed both Tami and Rob!

Mika later told me that she was truly worried I might jump over the edge of the ship, or demand halfway that I be returned to shore. I was that erratic and unreasonable.

The second memory I have was at lunchtime, when we were all supposed to meet Mika and Kai at a restaurant. I didn't want to see the older kids with their anxious eyes. So Rob went and I stayed back at the hotel with Tami and Matt, watching a movie instead. No interactions, no social competence, no sanity required. It was a welcome break from all the buzzing and butting of heads.

Third, in the afternoon, we went shopping in Chinatown. I normally hate shopping, but oh my, it was like I'd grown an extra pair of hands: I was grabbing unlikely items left and right, purchasing bright clothes I didn't even bother to try on and household items I would never use. The money flowed from my wallet as from a fountain. Uncharacteristic spending is a typical sign of hypomania, if only we'd known. I learned the hard way.

Before another train-wreck of a night, we decided to call my stepmom's brother, Sturla Bruun-Meyer, who's a psychiatrist in Toronto. I was still buzzy and exuberant, and he heard that in my voice immediately. But I wasn't altogether off the rails, so he just recommended an over-the-counter sleep medication to calm me down and help me sleep.

The minute I told Rob what Sturla had said, we did not walk, we *ran* to the nearest pharmacy! Poor Rob was desperate for some relief. He fully deserved it.

Mind you, so did I.

Niagara Falls

I did sleep a bit better that night – nothing spectacular, but more than the night before. Next morning, we drove to Niagara Falls with Jane, my friend from the pool. I couldn't wait to stand beside the Falls and in the gorge where the water rushes by, making seething waves more powerful than the ocean. I felt that the force of the water might somehow match my mental swirling; might pacify me. I was so excited by the prospect of visiting the Falls again that they tell me I jabbered incessantly all the way there. I was sitting in the back with Tami and Matt, and Jane and Rob were up front. At one point, Rob became so embarrassed by my rants that he reached behind him to squeeze my leg, as if to say: "Could you *please* give it a rest for a minute?" I was outraged. Who does he think he is? I'm doing nothing wrong! It seemed that whatever I said or did only earned disapproval or outright scorn from Rob. As if I could control myself!

Once we got to the Falls, things only degenerated. I felt totally misunderstood at every turn. I was just trying to arrange a fun visit for Jane and the kids, but whatever I did (buying entrance tickets, suggesting a place for lunch, chatting innocently to strangers on the tour bus, whatever) seemed to irritate or even exasperate Rob. Tami was distressed by Rob's and my constant bickering and felt sorry for Jane being stuck with us and having to pretend that she didn't notice the awkward tension. Rob and I normally never fight, so this was truly exceptional.

We finally got to my beloved gorge, and I walked alone, delighting in the fantastic force of the water. That is one of my favourite spots on earth, and I could have spent the whole day there, communing with the wild, raging river. At the end of the walkway, there's a lookout spot near some huge boulders. I clambered onto a high rock.

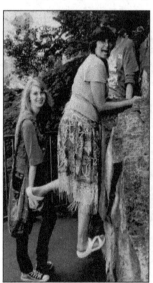

Climbing the rock at Niagara Falls; I have my wild-eyed and other-worldly look and face-splitting grin.

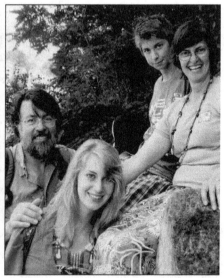

Rob (forcing a grimace-smile for the camera) and Tami standing; Matt and me up on the rock. I'm the only one having any fun at all. Classic hypomania!

Looking at the photos of me in action, I see that I really did look quite crazy.

Just after the second photo above was taken, I had an urge to take a photo of the swirling water from high up on the rock. I asked Rob to pass the camera up to me. Because of my over-excitement, I didn't pay proper attention and his very expensive camera slipped through my fingers, crashing onto the concrete path below. Even as it fell, I flashed back to Kai's laptop crashing to the asphalt just two days before. Again, I felt awful. Probably because Jane was with us, Rob reacted remarkably calmly to this incident. He later said he knew this was an accident caused by my racing pace.

Jane had to get back to Toronto for a meeting, so she left us soon after that to catch a bus.

Whew. I no longer had to keep up a pretense for her.

Rob later joked that he wished he could have just taken a bus and left, too!

He was having a truly awful time with me.

We headed back to the visitors' centre for lunch. But *en route*, I wanted to be spontaneous and take one of those novelty photos with the kids. I have never considered such a thing before: it always seemed too cheesy. Rob couldn't believe my antics and would have nothing to do with the whole project.

You get to choose a computer-generated background, and then you pose either in costume or doing something funny, and they combine the two images.

We chose to be Harry Potter-like, flying on broomsticks over the Falls. To make the flying look realistic, they had us jump high in the air and kick up our heels while perched on the brooms.

It was great fun.

The final photo is a priceless memento and a symbolic snapshot of the entire hypomanic episode. Both kids look wonderful, really having fun, and my hair is windswept from the jump and my mouth is wide open in a jubilant grin.

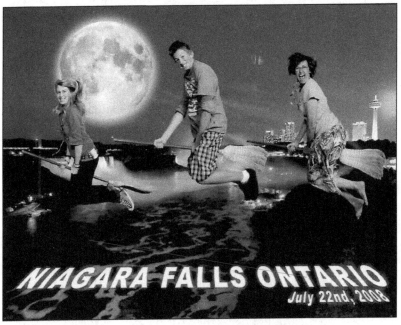

Tami, Matt and me: flying high over the Falls.
That's what this whole hypomanic episode felt like to me: glorious fun!

Choosing a place for lunch became another tussle between Rob and me. I wanted something quick from a fast food restaurant; he wanted a sedate sit-down meal in the fancy restaurant overlooking the Falls. Having seen the formal and slightly pretentious menu there, both kids sided with me. I impulsively stalked out of the restaurant, beckoning the kids to follow me. We could meet up with "old misery" later. Then, equally impulsively, I suggested that we drive to a tourist attraction where they simulate a skydive by blasting air into a room so that it lifts you off your feet and you feel like you're flying.

There's that flying theme again.

I'm not sure if it was my own idea to scrap that plan, or if Tami and Matt spoke some sense into me, but we all agreed that Rob would not be at all happy if I absconded, driving the minivan in my present state.

Oh. So there was a slight admission that there might be something a bit "off" with my mental state. But what? What on earth is happening to me, I wondered.

On second thought, just ignore that question. It was way too challenging to contemplate. And besides, I was having much too much fun to get serious just then.

Hamilton

That evening, July 22, we stayed with our old friends, Andy Orkin and Cheryl Levitt, in Hamilton. My mental state left an immediate impression on Andy: he later said it was clear to him within about thirty seconds of my arrival that I was mentally "out of whack" and utterly manic. He also said the kids were clearly shell-shocked, and Rob was exhausted.

While Rob, Andy and the kids were busy elsewhere, I jabbered to Cheryl, bitching about Rob's sudden unreasonableness towards me. I suppose that the mere speed of my speech clued her in. Being a family physician, she has seen it all at one time or another. She also knew about my earlier depression because Rob had called her for advice at the time. She says she remembers being quite overwhelmed, devastated and shocked by how different and manic I was and was immediately concerned that I had bipolar. She brought a cup of tea, sat down next to me, and calmly, matter-of-factly said: "You know, Merryl, you may have bipolar disorder."

Bipolar disorder.

I shuddered. I knew almost nothing about bipolar at the time but had once heard a woman say in hushed tones, while rolling her eyes: "Well, my husband has bipolar, you know. So I can't get out much…" Was I to become housebound and dependent on obligated caregivers? What might this mean?

My instinct was simply to resist it. What did Cheryl know, anyway? She had only seen me for about five minutes! I put her comment aside, buried it deep, and roared on through the evening. But I tried heroically to behave well throughout, needing to prove to myself and everyone else that I was, in fact, just fine.

At bedtime, I was feeling quite proud of myself. I expected Rob to soften after our tense interactions all day and say something kind about how well the evening had gone. No such luck. I had again unintentionally infuriated him, and after a few stinging words, he hissed: "You know, you're totally psychotic!"

Now I had him. At least I knew what psychotic meant, from my training as a nurse. I also knew that there was no good reason for him to know the actual meaning of the word. So it was clear that he was using it as an insult, merely trying to hurt me, and I became extremely defensive. I tried to humiliate him for using such a loaded word incorrectly: he should know better. When we both finally calmed down, we passed a decidedly frosty night in the guest bed, lying stiffly, back-to-back.

Despite the fight, I slept well and started the next day feeling much more composed and placid than the day before. It was as if an abscess had burst during the "psychotic" slur, and we were now both healing a bit.

Back home to Montreal

The drive back home was relatively uneventful, thanks again to iPoddy.

The Herzl Family Practice Centre at the hospital squeezed me in just two days later to be assessed for possible bipolar disorder. This time, I saw a different doctor because my original doctor (who diagnosed situational depression) was on vacation. We went over the whole history of the depression, and though I was still hypomanic, I think I was able to keep a lid on it for the duration of the interview. I came off as fairly sane. Unfortunately, this only delayed my referral to a psychiatrist, which is ultimately what I needed. Nevertheless, I was asked to return for another visit one week later. They clearly wanted to keep a close eye on me.

China plans

Imagine this: without consulting Rob or anyone else, I arbitrarily decided that our whole family should relocate to China. I printed out maps and tried to figure out which province and city would be best for us to move to. In my misfiring brain, we were all destined to live in China.

Within a week of taking Jane to Niagara, I emailed her to follow up and tell her that I hoped to see her in Beijing really soon. She responded politely, clearly doubting that my plans would materialize.

When I look back on this, I see how mad I must have been at the time, but I also see that there was a kernel of wisdom in planning at least a business trip to China. The smoking reduction work that Rob and I do with Indigenous communities in Canada has enormous potential for adaptation in China, where smoking rates are also extremely high. But that's precisely the trouble with hypomania: the lines between brilliantly inspired and outrageously improbable ideas become horribly blurred. Too often, what I considered to be ingenious, Rob harshly dismissed as outright ridiculous.

No wonder we rubbed each other the wrong way so much during hypomanic episodes.

(I don't remember this at all, but Tami tells me that in the same week I contacted Jane about relocating to China, I also emailed my school friend Phyllis in Australia to investigate the possibility of going to live there, too. Good grief.)

Road trip to Maine

In between my two appointments at the hospital and making my China plans, I spontaneously planned a road trip with Tami and Matt to drive to Maine in the United States, where Karrie was volunteering at a Baha'i summer camp for two weeks. (That's why she had been spared all the drama of our Toronto trip.)

She had arranged to get a lift home with another family, but I was still buzzing and restless after Toronto, and fancied the idea of taking a break from Rob for a few days.

Now, to understand the impact of hypomania on me, you need to know that I am normally quite content to let Rob drive, and to take in the scenery or the company without the stress of driving and navigating. I have never planned and executed a road trip in all my life. But this time, I researched beaches and hotels online, made the necessary bookings, got directions, organized snacks for the car, got the passports together, and so on. And all without feeling any stress.

The two kids and I then got in the van and happily headed south. We played loud music most of the way, stopped whenever we felt like it, and finally arrived, without a hitch, at our little beach hotel close to Karrie's camp. After a night in the hotel, we spent time on the beach and then in the arcade, trying all kinds of different games and activities. I was having fun, fun, fun!

After that, we met up with Karrie and headed north, stopping at Crescent Beach, Maine, on the way, and then spending a night in the New Hampshire mountains. Again, we found our way there with no problems, and had no unpleasant incidents *en route*. And so on, all the way home to Montreal. This little trip was a deeply empowering experience for me, and a great opportunity to bond with the children. However, if you asked me to replicate what I did then, now that I am stable, I would insist: "No way! Let's ask Rob to drive us!"

Follow-up clinic visit

At the next visit to the clinic at the hospital, the resident who had seen me initially and diagnosed situational depression decided that the clinical picture was in fact more complicated, and she referred me to a psychiatrist, Dr. Y. He gave me an appointment just twelve days later.

Dreaded diagnosis

My first appointment with Dr. Y involved a two-hour assessment, a half-hour phone call with Rob while I waited outside, and then a further half-hour discussion with me. Extremely thorough, but I was exhausted by the end of it all.

As it turns out, I was still hypomanic, and Dr. Y recognized it immediately. That, together with the history of a six-week depression shortly before caused him to confirm the dreaded diagnosis of bipolar. "You have a typical case of Bipolar Type II. You will need to be on lithium for life plus a short-term major tranquilizer until the lithium starts to work." That's what I remember him saying. (Please see Appendix 1 for definitions of Type I and Type II, etc.)

Dr. Y urged me to start treatment without delay, explaining that the longer you wait, the worse the condition can get. The brain gets used to misfiring, and next time there is an episode, it can be fiercer than before, going deeper for depression or higher for hypomania, and lasting longer. This is called the "kindling effect."

I wasn't ready to commit to medications, but I didn't tell Dr. Y that yet. I had a serious fear of meds and their side effects, and much preferred alternative therapies like acupuncture and naturopathy, coupled with talk therapy, yoga, meditation and relaxation.

Also, taking psychiatric medications would mean truly accepting the diagnosis. I was still in denial.

I'll never forget the feeling of utter desolation as I left Dr. Y's office that day. I walked deadpan down the corridor, fearing that I might encounter another patient or doctor, and they would see how devastated I was. I felt like someone had kicked me in the solar plexus, and I was gasping for air. My entire identity as a normal, sane, healthy, dependable adult had been shattered. My life would never be the same. And yet I was left to stagger, unescorted, uncared for, out of the building, onto the bustling street carrying the oppressive burden of this awful diagnosis; I was expected to get into the car and drive myself home as if nothing had happened in there. It felt surreal. I watched my every move in slow motion. And I observed the people around me, going on with their lives as if nothing had happened. I wanted to shriek at them: "Help me! He says I'm mad!"

Shell-shocked and disbelieving, I called Rob from the car. "He says I have bipolar." Numb. Wanting to fight it, but instinctively knowing that was probably pointless. "I can't believe it. This sucks so much."

Rob was gently empathetic; said he wished he were there to drive me home so I didn't have to be alone. But he later said he knew quite well by then that I had bipolar – from his research online, from Cheryl, and from when Dr. Y had called – so he wasn't at all shocked by my news. In fact, he was almost relieved: now that we know what's wrong, we can deal with it properly.

In late August, my friend Lida shared some helpful insights with me. Among other things, she said: "It's important to love ourselves regardless of the state we are in. We may like our healthy selves better, but we must be kind to ourselves and accept ourselves as we are, even when not feeling well. We may not be able to accomplish too much in a day, but it's better to focus on what we do accomplish. Patience is key. The healing journey is often long, and the support of family and friends makes all the difference. We just need to keep going until we feel better. This is not easy and requires a lot of courage and perseverance."

Sometime later, I began to see bipolar as a part of me, rather than an external problem. I began to accept it and accept myself with bipolar. I wondered: Is bipolar like a new marriage partner with whom I have to learn to dance?

Despite all my efforts to treat that first episode of hypomania, it continued from mid-July until mid-August 2008. It was a frenzied gallop through territory I never knew existed. Ninety percent of me enjoyed every minute of this episode: colours were more vivid, music more pleasing (perhaps this accounts for my unnatural emotional attachment to iPoddy?), experiences more exhilarating, and life in general was much more fun. The other ten percent was vaguely aware that my out-of-control behaviour was upsetting my family, and that I owed it to them to try to rein myself in.

But how to do that? I clearly needed help, but what kind?

Chapter 5: Getting help

At my first appointment with Dr. Y on August 13, 2008 when he handed me the dreadful diagnosis, he prescribed Risperdal 0.5mg four times a day for ten days only. I never filled that prescription. I was still giving alternative therapies a try.

At my second appointment with him, less than a week after he diagnosed me, I took a list of issues to discuss, and made notes about what he said. (His words appear in quotation marks below.)

1. I have definitely come down since my previous appointment. Rob now rates me as a 9.25 out of 10, where my normal rating is 9 out of 10. (I have always been an energetic, highly productive person.) But I do still feel mentally cloudy, not able to focus or work. "That's to be expected," he said.

2. Will there be a kindling effect if I delay onset of psychiatric meds? "Possibly; that is a risk."

3. "Triggers for you to go hypomanic seem to be sleep deprivation, stress and heavy workload. Things that could help control it include stress reduction, regular sleep, healthy food, and exercise."

4. I asked him about the advisability of my going away for a short retreat. "Only if you are supervised, as you might have another episode at any time. Now is not the ideal time. And beware: in hypomania and mania, people are exceptionally suggestible."

5. "Some people can get 'addicted' to hypomania."

6. "Don't make any big decisions while you are unstable." (Oh, like about relocating the family to China, for example?)

7. I asked for an appointment with a psychologist. "We don't recommend talk therapy until patients are stable. You could be referred to a psychologist at the hospital later on."

8. "The average length of a hypomania episode is twelve weeks, and depression, nineteen weeks."

9. "The main difference between hypomania and mania is that mania is often accompanied by psychosis and very dangerous behaviours."

10. "Bipolar is not a smooth progression of one high followed by one low and so on in a regular wave-like pattern. Rather, for most people, it goes either something like high, high, low, low, low, huge high, huge low, high, high... or small high, long flat, long low, flat, big high, flat, etc."

11. "The goal of lithium treatment now is to prevent future episodes (there is a 90% chance of recurrence if untreated; a 30% chance if treated) and to contain the extremes of any future episodes."

12. Dr. Y ended the appointment by listing the side effects of lithium: mental dullness, weight gain and acne being the commonest; may also get a fine tremor, thirst (and night-time urination), nausea, diarrhea, reversible hypothyroidism (5%), irreversible kidney damage (1%), and increased calcium in the blood.

A note to myself after this extremely informative appointment read:

Proceed AS IF the diagnosis is correct, just in case!

So I was still in denial, but softening. I have to credit Dr. Y's extreme politeness and patience with me: I felt respected and heard, and although I thought he must be exasperated by my reluctance to start on lithium, he was clearly willing to work with me through my fears. Scheduling frequent appointments kept me on a short leash and ultimately had the effect of slowly corralling me in.

Another note from the same day, addressed to Dr. Y but never shared, says:

> You should hand clients a list of relevant community organizations on the same day as their diagnosis. It took me a full week to do an online search, and I was in no fit state to be doing research about support groups etc. after the shock of the diagnosis and while still hypomanic...

I also made notes to myself to read up about bipolar in general, and about lithium in particular. (So, the softening continues. I was at least prepared to consider lithium as a treatment option.)

At the end of August, Tami and I went on a wonderful retreat together. We stayed at a luxury hotel nearby, where we swam in the indoor pool, lazed in the hot tub, sweated in the steam room, and then swam again to cool off. We ate in the excellent restaurant. We relaxed in our private Jacuzzi. We watched movies while lounging on our over-sized beds. We slept late. And we had hot stone massages in our suite. It was blissful. All this to calm and restore me after the hypomania in Toronto.

Four days later, Rob and I attended a meeting of the Depression and Bipolar Support Alliance (DBSA) West Island, which I'd discovered online. There was only a small group of participants that night, but it was shocking to hear people share their experiences. I didn't really relate to their horror stories, being so new to Bipolar Country myself, or feel ready to join the group. I was still in partial denial about my diagnosis, after all. But it was comforting to know that the group was there as a resource. Rob was appalled to hear the extent to which their mental illnesses had totally wrecked their lives: divorce; alienation from family members; bankruptcy; sex addiction; can't work...

A sobering night for us both.

My research had turned up another local community organization, Friends for Mental Health. There, Rob and I worked with an amazing counsellor, Lucy Lu, for about a dozen sessions over the next nine months. We found her to be gentle, insightful, skilled, caring and highly professional. My notes after the first meeting with her on September 5, 2008 say:

> Excellent! Very helpful and practical suggestions and interventions about managing stress and improving family dynamics and communication. Keep a daily log to rate my mood. Each of us must ask: How do I recharge my battery (e.g. introverts stay home; extroverts spend time with people)? She is open to complementary treatments. Not patronizing... I love her! She gave us lots of homework to read.

Lucy gave us a handout titled *Caregivers' Bill of Rights*, intended to highlight the needs of people like Rob, caring for mentally ill family members. I didn't miss a beat before insisting: "But we also need a *Mental Patients' Bill of Rights,* you know!" I took an extra copy of the handout to edit from my perspective as a patient. It felt wonderful to strike through, in forceful red pen, certain sections of the document, and add in phrasing that reflected my experience. In hindsight, a major source of stress was my dependence on Rob, and being the object of his and the children's caring concern. That wasn't the way it was supposed to be: *I* was supposed to care for and worry about *them.* So the *Caregivers' Bill of Rights* felt somewhat patronizing to me, as if I were such a burden being the "loved one" of my "caregiver," Rob. This sanitized language annoyed me at the time: I was Rob's wife, that's all. Not his "loved one." And he was my husband, not my "caregiver"…

In sickness and in health, remember?

One week later, during our second session, Lucy diagnosed a problem in the communication between Rob and me, and she gave us homework to mirror back for five minutes each day to ensure that we had truly heard each other. "I heard you say that …" or "I feel … when …" She said: "You need to lower the temperature of your relationship." That was so helpful. She also gave us a *Contract for the treatment of bipolar disorder* which specified what I should do if I felt that I needed help at any time (e.g. ask Rob to call a doctor or take me to hospital, etc.). There was a *Family Crisis Plan* on the back of the contract, with blank spaces to fill in phone numbers for my mental health professional, the police, a trusted relative or friend, and so on. The idea was to be well-prepared in case a crisis struck.

There were continuing residual angry spikes between Rob and me despite our best efforts to keep the peace. Rob still found me too hypomanic on occasion. I was committed to my naturopathic remedies, but Rob was getting impatient with the lack of response. He wanted me on "proper treatment." The pressure was building. I felt he was siding with Dr. Y, not me!

In our third session with Lucy, on September 26, she advised: prioritize your lives and the various commitments you have, so you can live more sustainably; conserve energy – do things to a level of "just good enough" rather than perfection (as both Rob and I were guilty of); limit yourselves to eight hours a day to earn a living, to leave time for volunteer activities, rest and relaxation; and recognize that coping with bipolar disorder sucks up an enormous amount of energy, especially in the early stages.

In between all this, I had seen Dr. Y on August 26 and September 23. At that time, he scheduled my fifth appointment for October 20, but that was brought forward by two weeks to October 7 because I went into another mind-numbing depression on October 4. That depression was the final wake-up call I needed to convince me that Dr. Y's diagnosis (and Cheryl's, some months before) was, unfortunately, perfectly accurate.

To everyone's relief, I finally agreed to take lithium.

Dr. Y started me on a dose of 300mg twice a day, and one week later at my sixth appointment, he checked blood levels of lithium and increased the dose to 300mg plus 600mg daily. This dose was maintained at my seventh visit the following week when he again checked blood levels. My notes indicate that although my appetite had improved, there was "zero mood lifting." The depression had settled in with a dogged determination. Dr. Y said it usually takes from two to four months to recover from a depressive episode. Good grief; this is my life passing here!

At around this time, on October 10 – our fourth meeting with Lucy – she prescribed a "date" for Rob and me: for three hours, just the two of us, leaving the "third wheel" called bipolar at home. We were to report back to her next time. We chose to spend our date in the Morgan Arboretum, a peaceful oasis of woods near our home where we had gone walking, jogging, skiing and tobogganing since our first year in Canada. It was teeming with wonderful memories, and the trees were in full fall plumage, giving off a radiant energy that I sorely needed to absorb. Part of Lucy's prescription had been that each of us should be blindfolded for ten minutes, trusting our partner to lead us around safely and to end up at a special place that would say something about how we felt about each other. Rob blindfolded me and holding me tightly, tenderly led me to a beautiful birch, one of my favourite tree species. When he removed the blindfold, he noted how pleasing and elegant the birch was, and straight and true, just like you-know-who.

I then blindfolded Rob, and I led him to a much-loved old tree that the kids had played and posed in many times (see photo below) because it has multiple low-slung branches curving upwards like welcoming arms.

I positioned Rob directly in front of the trunk, and it looked like the branches were his many arms: strong, protective, sheltering, and well qualified to take care of me, regardless of what bipolar might throw at us. Unexpectedly, I began to weep. That image of Rob standing by the tree was such a perfect metaphor for his resolute support of me. When I explained why I was crying, Rob gave me a reassuring bear hug in the shade of our special tree. I remember that date with great affection.

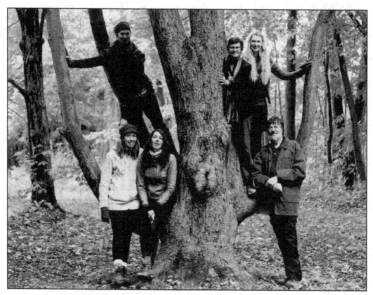

This photo from 2016 shows the much-loved tree I led Rob to.
L: Karrie & Mika with Matt above. R: Rob with me & Tami above.

For our fifth meeting with Lucy a week later, on October 17, I was still in depression, but not as deeply as before. We discussed our date and the insights we had both had from the blindfolding exercise, the benefits of a weekly date, keeping daily charts (see Appendix 2), and potential triggers for my depression. Lucy also suggested that I keep a personal journal to reflect on my reactions to myself, others, and bipolar.

As homework after that session, I made a mood chart for how I was feeling coming out of depression. The symptoms list read:

> Appetite returning; sleep a bit better (not good yet); can plan menus and shop for groceries; can start thinking about work (not yet *doing* work, though); can cope with social engagements (not yet the 'life

and soul of the party' though); lighter mood – can smile again; feel a bit hopeful; still hard to focus; not longing for bedtime all day; posture is upright with head held higher.

October 24 was our sixth meeting with Lucy, a week after the previous one. I was still stuck in that in-between place coming out of depression, but not yet out. My notes say:

> Lots of tears today. I can't work… feel guilty about Rob having to do it all. I don't know what to expect about the future.

Lucy challenged me to ask: "Who am I? Not just a person with bipolar; not just my work; then who?" We talked about the impact of my moods on the children: I was concerned that my depression might drag them down. Rob said he was not worried, either way: "We'll cope." That was majorly reassuring. He was so amazing when I went down, especially. Then Lucy said I should hold my emotions "like a baby, with tenderness and care." She said I wouldn't lock a crying baby in a room or blame the baby. I must learn to accept this "baby" of overwhelming emotions.

Radical thought.

My eighth visit to Dr. Y was on October 31. My blood level was 0.9, which he assured me was perfect. He said he found me "virtually back to normal" – eating, sleeping, good energy, coping in many aspects of life, but just not at work. He said he thought I had burnout, and that my current actions (baking apple pie, cooking, cleaning, etc.) were saying that I just wanted to be a wife and mother for now. (Most uncharacteristic!) "It will take time to get back into work mode; don't fight it." He said he'd complete the forms for disability insurance, so I could relax a bit about the major financial implications of this disorder.

Ten days later, on my fifty-second birthday on November 10, 2008, I saw Dr. Y for the ninth time. He handed me the completed insurance forms, which said he expects "full recovery" in four to six weeks. (That felt like a long shot to me.) He suggested that I do a half-day trial in the next two weeks, just to see if I could go into my office and focus for a few hours. Sensing that I was despondent about my inability to work, he tried to comfort me by saying he was treating lawyers, doctors, nurses, all kinds of high-functioning professionals who have bipolar. "It's quite possible to have both a productive career and bipolar disorder," he reassured.

Good to know.

My tenth appointment with Dr. Y was two weeks later in late November. Once again, I had made a list of issues to discuss with him. What worried me most was what I called "circular thoughts" and "mental distractions." Instead of sleeping, I would lie there and think of a specific event or something someone had said. Then an image or word from that would jump out and form a loop in my brain. There was one example around the word "partner." Someone had called her spouse "my partner," and that reminded me that in the dedication to my doctoral thesis I had referred to Rob as my partner. Then I had to remember all kinds of other details first about the thesis, then about the research leading up to it and all the people involved, then about a current research project of thesis-like proportions, and before you knew it, there went at least an hour or two of beauty sleep. (Or should I say: "sanity sleep"?) Dr. Y suggested that I try mindfulness meditation to stop these kinds of obsessive thoughts and redirect my mind to the present moment. Luckily, there are endless resources about mindfulness on YouTube. I highly recommend them.

Another issue I raised with Dr. Y was my detailed to-do lists and the pride I took in crossing off items. "This is probably just a coping mechanism to give you some sense of control. Your obsessive tendencies and perfectionist's attention to detail might account for the lists. And you might be seeking approval." I also told him that I still had an atypical interest in cleaning, tidying, baking, interior decorating – anything but intellectual work. He smiled knowingly and murmured as he made a note in my file: "So the boycott of office work continues, I see." He said maybe all the housework was a repackaged way to be helpful to the family, or maybe it sprang from regret that I hadn't done enough of that kind of work in the past.

He then said: "We may need to adjust your medications to get you functioning at 100%."

The seventh session with Lucy was the first one where I went alone: Rob was travelling for work. I was now – thankfully! – out of depression but mentioned that I was having some flares of anger that might indicate early signs of (hypo)mania.

Lucy recommended that I write a letter to myself committing to no more than eight hours of work per day, no high-risk volunteer work (i.e. where I get over-invested or -emotional), and generally undertaking to slow down and take good care of myself. She suggested that I do some online research, which I did.

As for the letter to myself, I decided to write a letter to Rob instead:

December 4, 2008.

Dearest Robby,

Lucy asked me to write a letter to myself to capture some of the promises I need to keep to maintain balance and stability – as much as is possible with bipolar… But I have chosen to write to you instead.

That way, I make the commitments to you as well as to myself. Also, I hope you will be able to buy in to the changes I am proposing to make. Of course, I'd love for you to join me on most of these items, but I also respect that you will make your own decisions, and I understand that you must be feeling enormous pressure to make up for the lost time that my illness has caused you and our consultancy over the past many months. However, I think we have all learned that energy is finite, and your turn to crash – either physically or mentally or both – will not be far off if you don't seek balance in your life as well. There; lecture over!

From what I've heard from both Lucy and Dr. Y, and from what I've read, I believe that the following changes would be beneficial for me to avoid my known triggers such as stress, exhaustion, emotional over-investment, concern for exceptional productivity, perfectionism, etc. See what you think!

OLD, WORKAHOLIC LIFESTYLE	NEW, BALANCED, HEALTHY LIFESTYLE
Work 12–14 hours/day routinely.	Work 8 hours/day maximum; use evening time to help the kids, cook, tidy, clean, relax, exercise, etc.
Everything seems to be a crisis that needs to be fixed immediately; every email is urgent and has to be responded to; etc.	Keep things in perspective; be realistic about what can be done in a day; relax! Ask: "Is this a medical emergency?"

Check emails every few minutes, interrupting other work in order to appear so efficient and professional.	Check emails once per hour maximum; only read urgent ones immediately; save the rest for later in the day when project work is done.
Perfectionist & obsessive about work: everything has to be perfect.	Lower my standards to "just good enough"; ask: "Is this worth making myself sick over?"
Little time for the children.	Make more time for the children; enjoy spending time with them doing whatever they want to do (homework, crafts, sports, music, etc.).
Very little time for friends; feel guilty taking time off to relax with friends.	Nurture my friendships; be emotionally available to others who have been so supportive of me when I needed them.
No hobbies.	Think about cultivating a relaxing hobby. Knitting? Piano? Hiking.
For long periods, exercise rarely or never, then "get back on the wagon" periodically.	Exercise regularly, consistently, at least 3 or 4 times per week; do yoga for flexibility and to reduce stress and relax.
Skip meals or pay no attention to eating when too busy with work (and when hypomanic).	Eat regularly; balanced meals; healthy choices.
Love to volunteer: get carried away with whatever the topic of the day is. Love to start new organizations from scratch, becoming emotionally invested in them, overwhelming time commitment.	Limit volunteer work to what is already on my plate. No extra responsibilities for at least 6 months. Reassess capacity at that stage, and decide in consultation with you if I can reasonably take on more, or if I want to switch from current commitments to new ones, etc.
Housework is neglected: do only the bare minimum in between blitzes when guests are coming.	Do housework regularly; try to approach it with a zen attitude.

Rarely cook/bake: special occasions only.	Pay more attention to cooking and baking. See this as a different way to be creative.
No time for dates or energy to nurture our marriage.	Weekly date with you; explore new ways of relaxing together: we both need that!
Go to sleep really late (1 or 2 a.m.; 3 or 4 a.m. on weekends).	Sleep at 11:30 p.m. latest every night, weekends included.
Get about 5 or 6 hours of sleep.	Get at least 8 hours of sleep.
Reject conventional medicine; prefer alternative therapies.	Take bipolar meds as prescribed.

The day after I wrote this letter, Rob and I saw Lucy for the eighth time. I was feeling almost back to normal. We mainly discussed my letter to Rob, which they both liked a lot.

A few weeks later, I adapted my letter to Rob into a chart titled *Maintain balance and stability as much as possible with bipolar: How am I doing these days?* I removed the paragraphs addressed to Rob and just wrote a brief introduction about reducing triggers and added a third column to this table titled *Rating out of 10* where I rated myself on each item before each visit to Lucy using a scale of 1–10 where 10 is excellent. It was hugely helpful to monitor myself so closely, and it really kept me on the straight-and-narrow regarding my commitments. It's not easy to reform oneself from being a workaholic, but with bipolar breathing down my neck, that was all the motivation I needed. I encourage you to make your own Balanced Life Chart with relevant items and a rating scale to help you avoid your own triggers.

On December 8, two weeks after my previous appointment, I saw Dr. Y for our eleventh appointment. I told him that there had been a big improvement concerning my "boy-cott" or resistance to work since the last visit. I gave him con-crete examples of the kind of work I had managed (mainly editing and proof-reading, plus attending two meetings with Rob), and said I had spent time in my office filing, tidying, sorting, and making a list – another list! – of priorities after a seven-month hiatus. "I don't dread going into my office any longer. I almost look forward to getting in there..." Dr. Y suggested a "progressive return to work": work for a total of four half-days over two weeks, then six half-days over the next two weeks, then eight half-days over the last two weeks.

I told Dr. Y that I was being extremely disciplined about bedtime, exercise, yoga, meditation, healthy meals, do-ing something relaxing in the evenings, not getting over-tired, and taking my meds religiously. A model patient, I thought!

I then asked if he would have any objection to my going on a three-week trip to the Arctic region of the Northwest Territories (NWT) with Rob to work on our research project there. He said it would be fine for me to go as long as I got enough sleep during the trip, and he cautioned that it gener-ally takes a day to adjust for each time zone difference.

Finally, I asked Dr. Y if it was possible that I had been hypomanic during the family crisis when I was so highly fo-cused, productive and buzzy while fighting for our child. He said yes, each episode can look remarkably different. So it seems that during the crisis in April and May, I was experi-encing a "hypomanic workaholic episode," but in Toronto, Niagara and Maine, it was a "hypomanic party episode."

Before leaving for the NWT trip, I felt nervous and in-secure. What if I have an episode while we're travelling? End-less "what ifs" eventually caused a mini-slump where my mood ratings dropped to 5 out of 10 and stayed low for five days. Rob was confident that I could handle this trip and encouraged me to commit to it. Within a day or two of me finally deciding it would be safe enough to go, we booked the air tickets and my mood lifted. I had a sense of purpose and felt responsible and competent, rather than indecisive and inept.

On January 12, 2009, I had my twelfth visit with Dr. Y. I had just returned from our successful trip to NWT, and told him: "Right now, I'm back; I am myself again." I was still monitoring my work schedule closely, but felt "100% focused, productive and creative." It was fantastic! I said I felt worthy again, and "normal." I told him that a day after my previous appointment with him in early December, I had a brief, mild depression and asked him if there was a name for such a mini-episode. "A 'depressive blip.' A true depressive episode lasts at least two weeks. On the other hand, you might also experience a brief 'hypomanic blip' whereas a true hypomanic episode lasts a minimum of four days."

I told him that I had another short business trip to Toronto coming up towards the end of January. I felt fine to go – even though Rob would not be accompanying me this time.

Dr. Y informed me that he now felt ready to discharge me back to the Herzl clinic after one last appointment in February. I felt deeply insecure at the thought. I couldn't imagine trusting a family medicine resident – or a series of rotating residents! – the way I trusted Dr. Y.

Our next meeting with Lucy was four days later, on January 16, 2009. As mentioned, I was functioning normally, and my mood was neither too high nor too low. I told her about my recent depressive blip that had been caused by ambivalence over my readiness to travel, and Lucy wondered whether indecision might not be a trigger for some of my depressions. She challenged me to think about how I manage uncertainty. (Being a control freak must surely make uncertainty a high-stress situation.) She also suggested that pressure to perform to a very high standard may also be a trigger. And guilt that Rob has to cover for me at work and at home.

On February 9, 2009, I saw Dr. Y for our thirteenth and final scheduled appointment. He gave me my latest blood results, all of which were fine. I had some questions about how lithium interacts with other drugs, for example anaesthetics ("There is a risk of delirium; go off lithium two days before elective surgery"); analgesics like Demerol and morphine ("Morphine is okay, but with Demerol there is a risk of serotonin syndrome – a potentially life threatening drug reaction – causing convulsions among other things"); decongestants for colds and flu ("Dextromethorphan – a cough suppressant used in many over-the-counter remedies – can cause serotonin syndrome; check with a pharmacist before taking anything"); and anti-malarials ("3 or 4 per 1,000 have a psychotic episode").

Note to self: don't take *any* other meds, ever!

I showed him my latest daily self-care chart and said it had been a great month. (I kept – and have continued to keep for many years after I finally became stable – a daily record of my moods, activities, sleep and medications; please see Appendix 2 for details.) He was well pleased. I told him that the trip to Toronto had been a big test for me, going without Rob, and I was proud that I had managed it. I was officially back to work full-time, since January 26, 2009, and we had informed the insurance company of this.

I then asked what additional meds I would need if I went either hypomanic ("Seroquel or Risperdal") or depressed ("Lamictal or Seroquel"). Just covering all the bases. "Highs are easier to treat than lows, but most family physicians are more scared of the highs, if only because they are rarer than lows."

Not to mention the bizarre behaviour the highs induce!

Dr. Y then carefully outlined my options at the Herzl clinic should anything go wrong: make an appointment at the Herzl; go to the walk-in clinic; go for a scheduled walk-in visit in the evening; or in a major crisis, go directly to the emergency. He said I could always recommend that they check with him about how best to proceed.

It was with real sadness that I thanked Dr. Y for all his months of respectful and understanding care. It really was "care" that he had provided, in every sense of the word. And so ended an era.

Almost.

After my first full-blown manic episode a few months later in the spring of 2009, Rob and I again met with Dr. Y for over two hours on June 9. In view of the pattern of recurring episodes that had emerged, he revised my diagnosis from Bipolar Type II to Bipolar Type I, rapid cycling. (Bipolar I involves periods of depression and full-blown mania, and rapid cycling bipolar involves four or more episodes of depression and/or (hypo)mania per year. Please see Appendix 1 for more definitions.) I requested a referral to the Douglas Mental Health University Institute (the Douglas) that – as its name implies – specializes in mental health issues and is closer to our home. I was assessed at the Evaluation Module at the

Douglas on July 15 and was immediately accepted as a patient in their bipolar unit.

~   ~   ~

During the same months that we worked with Lucy and I saw Dr. Y, from summer 2008 to early 2009, I explored many other potential resources, desperately hoping to shore up enough support to prevent further ups and downs.

I tried naturopathy, mindfulness, yoga, nutrition therapy, and massage therapy. I consulted a second naturopath who specialized in orthomolecular approaches, which aim to combine orthomolecular solutions (such as vitamin and mineral supplements) with mainstream psychiatric medications (chemical solutions) to reduce the dose of chemicals required, but not to eliminate them. I ordered books and did numerous Internet searches about bipolar and the various treatments I was put on. One month, I ordered five self-help books about bipolar. It goes without saying, this was overwhelming, and all five sat unread on the shelf for many, many months before I was in any fit state to study them. But I felt more secure just knowing they were in the house. It was a major-time job for me to contact all these resource people and do all the associated research, often when I was feeling far from competent, but I instinctively knew that if I didn't seek help, I would continue flailing helplessly and would eventually sink.

Bipolar is a complex brute, so you need a multi-pronged approach to control it.

You can see that I reached out for help in as many places as I could think of. My old workaholic tendencies took over, and I researched bipolar and its treatments and support systems as thoroughly as possible.

Anything that seemed reasonable to me, I tried.

I remember what Dr. Y had warned: "Beware: in hypomania, people become exceptionally suggestible." I longed for a magic potion that would return me to my pre-bipolar state and undo the damage I had done to my brain. In my desperate search for a solution, I sometimes completely suspended disbelief. But there is no magic potion.

Stability has to be earned and learned, step-by-step, day-by-day. At first, I was looking for external resources to save me. I now know that I have to do the work, every day, myself.

I also reached out to far-away family and friends for emotional support. You cannot imagine the feelings of unworthiness and shame that the diagnosis of a mental illness had caused me. I knew intellectually that I was not at fault, but I judged myself nonetheless. I had internalized the stigma around mental illness. Having the acceptance of others was priceless.

In all the above ways, I tried to reach out for help. Grasping at straws in some cases; finding meaningful assistance and support in others. And before I would reach the safe harbour of stability, I had to endure many more episodes of highs and lows.

Despite my best efforts to keep the bipolar beast tamed using both conventional and alternative therapies, she raged on with unrelenting fury, totally taking over my life.

As I said, it was in the spring of 2009 that I had my first full-blown manic episode and Dr. Y had to revise his initial diagnosis.

Mania deserves a chapter – or two! – of its own.

Chapter 6: Mania starts

Before my first true manic episode, I endured another severe depression which ironically began immediately after a session with a mindfulness coach in April 2009. Walking to my car afterwards, I felt that old familiar dark veil coming down. It flapped around me menacingly, and I furiously tried to shake it off, striding more determinedly, head up, shoulders back, desperately trying to "walk-and-talk" myself out of it. But as I drove home, it settled around me like a stifling black hood. I had never before felt the start of a depressive episode in such a palpable, physical way. I felt devastated: oh no; here we go again…

In May, after five weeks of that wretched episode, I emerged, hoping for at least a couple of weeks of stability. No such luck. My notes indicate that I went into my office after many weeks of not working and did some good work. Then I went for a brisk walk with Tami. I wrote:

Amazing day!! I'm back!!

Liberal use of exclamation marks is always a warning that hypomania is looming.

Just the next morning I added:

Yikes – couldn't sleep at all: must be a bit hypomanic. That means a "switch" directly from depression to hypomania in one day! Talk about "rapid cycling"!

Did good work till nearly 3:30 a.m., then watched
the sunrise before going to bed. Woke at 8 a.m. Feeling great – not tired; not irritable (yet)!

On the next day, I wrote:

Great day, but there were several squabbles with
Rob caused by my irritability and his judgmental-
ness. At the party tonight, I was confident, sociable,
the "life and soul" – chatting, laughing, even singing. I sat far from Rob. He looked miserable. Men!

On the following day, I noted:

BUZZING all day and madly irritable. Huge fight
with Rob during which he kind of "restrained" my
arm. Argh! And he used his foot to try to block my
way out of the room. How *dare* he? ZERO hours
sleep.

Things were so bad we called the Herzl clinic and they consulted with Dr. Y who prescribed Risperdal in addition to
lithium.

The next day, the two girls became the object of my
wrath for some reason. I snarled: "I could throttle both of
you!" To which Karrie calmly replied: "In five minutes you'll
regret saying that." And to which Tami retorted: "Well, we
could throttle *you!*"

My brain fired off red-hot flares, fireworks and missiles.
I was only dimly aware that my family was in grave danger of
being shot down by my vitriolic verbal attacks, uncharacteristic actions, and unpredictable mental explosions that seared,
exasperated and exhausted them all.

It felt like my brain had become a volcano that violently coughs and splutters, spewing deadly lava like dreadful hot sputum from the depths of the earth's diseased lungs. The toxic lava merged into fiery ribbons and coursed downhill, scorching and flattening everything in its path. The eruptions had blinding force, thrusting skyward in all directions. These natural pyrotechnics were breathtaking but terrifying. There was a fierce dragon in there, spitting mad, out of control.

By coincidence, my friend Phyllis in Australia emailed me some amazing footage of Mount Etna erupting. I gushed:

> Spectacularly amazing!! I LOVE it. OK, now imagine: that's exactly how my brain felt this weekend. I am spiking a major high episode: sleep zero hours all night, then nap for two hours at 8 a.m. if I'm lucky...
>
> Recently, I went for over forty hours without sleep. I have become really irritable with Rob and the kids...
>
> It will pass. This brain eruption will end.
>
> But what damage will have been done?
>
> And where will the lava land?

As I mentioned in the *Prologue*, it was sometime during the ecstatic torment of all this drama that I had the idea to capture all these moments and share them in a book. This, of course, is the book that I imagined.

Despite the psychological chaos I was lost in during this episode, I wrote copious notes, mainly jotted hurriedly on post-its that I saved in a big pile. I also kept my old agenda that lists appointments and other commitments. Both these sources have enabled me to accurately re-live many of my experiences during the wildly tumultuous weeks of mania – which I was still mistakenly referring to as hypomania at the time.

Why did I feel the need to keep detailed notes even at the height of the episode?

Perhaps it was force of habit from my academic and nursing training, where records have to be accurate and complete for future reference.

Or perhaps pinning down my frantically whizzing thoughts on paper made me feel at least some self-possession and control, some small sense of mastery in an otherwise out-of-control drama – something I sorely needed in that frazzled state.

And, as I said, I had the idea, somewhere in the back of my deeply distressed mind, that I would one day write a book about all this, and I knew I'd need material for that.

My thoughts were speeding so fast (what psychiatrists refer to as "flight of ideas"), I used the analogy of racehorses galloping past to explain to my family how it felt. Each racing idea seemed critically important to lasso (to capture by scribbling it down), and I was irrationally emotionally attached to each one. If I didn't catch it immediately as it charged past, it would be lost forever. To be sure, another racehorse/idea would follow just behind, but I desperately wanted to lasso *this* one. *Now!*

When an idea inevitably eluded me, I got so frustrated and agitated it often reduced me to wailing tears.

I kept post-its and pens in every available place: in my purse, in all the rooms of the house where I was likely to be, even in the washroom and taped to the tiled wall where I lay in the bath, trying to calm myself. I just couldn't bear to miss a brilliant idea that might charge by at an inconvenient moment. I had no control over when the ideas would come; all I could do was be ready to trap them as they sped past.

The more manic I became, the more post-its I scribbled each day. I even wrote post-its about post-its. For example, I rather smugly noted that in a single day "I wrote 32 post-its excluding this one." One post-it read: "Take photo of post-its!" So a small part of my misfiring brain was still functioning logically. I knew that a photo would be a good reminder for me, and possibly a good image to include in this book. (Unfortunately, the photo I did take was very poor quality, so it's not included here.)

Some post-its had only one idea, but some had several ideas squished onto them with writing going in all directions. I was scrawling so fast my writing was barely legible at times.

Some listed things to do, such as "Order bipolar book online," while others were more creative – and ambitious! – like: "Make a movie about a menopausal woman with bipolar." I even fantasized about having my favourite actress, Meryl Streep, playing the leading role. Another post-it from the same evening says: "Huge creative storm! While watching *Slumdog Millionaire* with the kids, I filled six large post-its."

So many thoughts, so many new ideas, so much creative energy. My head felt like an over-inflated balloon about to explode.

It felt there were piercing spikes and red-hot light sabres sticking out of my brain. There were times I was so distraught and overwhelmed by the raging flood of ideas that I had to call Tami or Rob to "play secretary" for me. I would either lie on the bed, thrashing feverishly, or spin on a swivel chair while barking out random, disconnected thoughts that they would jot down as fast as possible – never fast enough to keep up with my bolting brain.

Quite a scene.

After a storm of ideas like that, my exhausted brain would finally change gears or even totally stall for a while. Then I would play some music or watch something on YouTube while I rested. But even then, I still didn't need to sleep.

Sometimes I forgot that I had already written a post-it about a specific topic and would scrawl the same idea a day or two later, believing it to be an original thought. Given the swirling storm in my brain, it's surprising this didn't happen more often, since I wasn't referring back to my notes at all at the time; I felt much too wired and crazed to do that. In fact, all those post-its and other notes stayed in untended piles for two full years before I ever looked at them again, in preparation for writing this book. What a vivid trip back in time they provided.

I guess part of me was embarrassed to re-live the "post-it days" too soon after the drama they so accurately captured.

My main emotion during this time was elation. I was buzzing, fizzing, whizzing, bubbling, whirling like a dervish. But I also felt judged, patronized, irritable, angry, steaming, boiling, furious, isolated, confused, terrified and self-centred. I was unusually creative, and felt mysteriously in tune with nature.

I remember one night feeling intensely squirmy and anxious, as though not just my head but my whole body was going to lift up off the bed and float away. I yelled for Rob to lie on top of me to pin me down. "Help me!" I sobbed. "Hold me down harder!"

A few days into this manic crisis, Rob and I were unduly prickly with each other, like in Toronto and Niagara, only way worse. He was always so understanding and patient with me when I was depressed, but unforgiving and judgmental – or so it seemed to me – when I went up. As if I were in control of my mood; my behaviour!

Didn't he know that my brain was a tsunami, smashing onto the shore and sweeping away everything in its path?

In a huff after one particularly testy interaction with him, I had a brilliant idea: I'm going to move down into the basement guest room so I don't have to deal with his negative vibes all day long. (We both work from home, so it's impossible to escape each other.)

Before disappearing downstairs, I researched what might be happening in my brain during (hypo)mania. I found brain scan images on the Internet of people with (hypo)mania and with depression. In (hypo)mania the brain is lit up joyfully, indicating excessive neuronal firing, and in depression the brain is almost entirely dark, devoid of cognitive functioning.

How apt. And how comforting to see that there is objective, physical evidence to support what I was feeling subjectively.

Another image of bipolar showed a brain with firing blue sparks coming out of it at all angles. That one spoke to me so clearly I printed a large colour copy of it, pasted it onto cardboard, made a string necklace, and hung it around my neck to remind my family: "I have bipolar. Don't blame me."

My head felt like it had exploded and I had pulsating neurons protruding from my skull like an Afro hairdo. And the Afro was dyed in flashy, rainbow colours.

I guess that's why I found headscarves and hats so reassuring: they seemed to "contain" my unruly neurons; keep them somewhat in check.

I chose the most colourful scarf I could find and draped it flamboyantly over my racing head.

In this elaborate getup, then, I excitedly exiled myself to the basement.

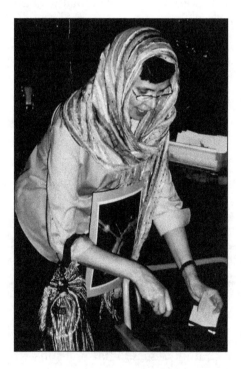

Relocating to the basement, scribbling post-its even as I went. A headscarf (or hat) soothed me. The graphic of a "manic brain" hanging around my neck is to remind my family members of my frantic mental state. (As if they needed reminding!)

Down in the basement, I had great fun playing house, re-organizing and re-decorating the 12' x 12' guest room to create a private little haven for myself and my new best buddy, mania. Even in that frenzied state, it struck me as odd that this was giving me so much pleasure: I never normally have any interest in interior design.

By re-arranging the furniture, I created "an office," "bedroom," "dining room" with a chair and a tray for dishes, "sitting room," "music room" for my guitar, and a "gym" where my yoga mat squeezed beside the bed. I re-decorated the bathroom just down the hall with candles, ornaments, fancy soaps and a satisfying selection of bright post-its. Rob and the children kept me well fed and when no one was around, I occasionally crept upstairs to help myself to food, which I then took down to my private "dining room" to eat in peace.

I avoided contact with the whole family as much as possible – less chance of friction.

Not only did I re-arrange furniture, I tried to beautify my temporary little home. I draped vivid hand-printed fabrics from Africa all over, displayed many ornaments from upstairs, and even placed fake flowers in the window-well outside so that when I looked out I'd see something bright and appealing. No amount of vibrancy or gaudiness could satisfy my craving for brilliant colours and bold designs.

After a busy day of re-organizing, I had created a true refuge for myself. I felt secure, content, and proud of what I had accomplished. I thought I'd never want to leave.

Feeling momentarily magnanimous, I invited the family down to see the transformation and to visit what I thought of as either my "Retreat Room" or, jokingly, the "Locked Ward," depending on how I felt at the time. Bad mistake. No one seemed at all impressed with my amazing achievements!

Hrmph.

My notes from that day say:

This room is the BEST idea ever!! Peace and quiet;
no one to fight with or growl at. And no one to judge
or blame me. Whew! What a relief! They can all go
to hell!

Mika heard about my voluntary relocation via the family
grapevine and emailed her strong approval from Toronto.
Perhaps channelling Virginia Woolf, she wistfully mused that
everyone should be so lucky as to have a "room of one's own."

Of course, Woolf meant a room for a woman to think
and write in, whereas I needed a room to be magnificently
mad in.

That night, Rob sent a frugal email with the subject
line: "I love you." The message itself was just three words: "I
mean it!" Very sweet.

I wanted to strictly control any potential traffic to my
new sanctuary. So I made three colourful signs to place outside my door depending on my mood.

The first sign was perfectly simple:

Kindly knock before entering. Thanks.

The second one read:

Please do NOT knock. Open my door VERY,
VERY QUIETLY to see if I'm sleeping or not. If I
am, please let me catch up on some much-needed
sleep! ZZZZZZ.

The third sign said:

Please DO NOT DISTURB: sleeping or writing potentially important thoughts! I'll remove this sign when I'm awake or less occupied. Thank you for your patience and understanding. P.S. I love you!

As it happened, almost no one except Tami (and Rob – mainly when I called for him in a frenzy to help me lasso race-horses) came downstairs at all. People were either fearful of me, or they really respected my need for privacy and peace. Or both.

I had fun using the three signs and thought what a shame it was that I was really the only one who saw them at all. But the calm was critical for me, so it's just as well the family left me largely to myself.

Several uncharacteristic interests and pastimes emerged during this manic episode:

1. Want to get a facial: got one in early June. This was my first-ever professional facial.

2. Want massages: had several during this episode. I never normally go for massages.

3. Buy new clothes and accessories. Fashion is normally about the last thing on my mind.

4. Consider highlights for my hair. This would have been out of the question in my normal state: too frivolous for me!

5. Wear make-up at all times. Normally, I wear none.

6. Want to go back to school to study neuropsychology.

7. Sudden new interests in: woodwork, architecture, interior design, landscape design, gardening.

8. Inventions: I have never been inventive in any technical way. But during this episode it was as if a whole new part of my brain suddenly came online and I could design inventions that seemed to me to be worthy of patenting.

The same day that I moved into my retreat room and the day after, I thought that we should print cards and T-shirts with clever slogans to help break down the stigma of bipolar. After I had made a list of 24 ideas, I wrote:

> To cater to all tastes, we need some humourous, some a bit outrageous, some subtle, some sentimental, etc.

Here's a sample:

1. *(Front)* Please forgive me… *(Back)* I have bipolar and honestly can't control myself at times.

2. *(Front)* If you think this is bad… *(Back)* You should see me when I forget my meds.

3. *(Front)* I know I exasperate you when I have mood swings. *(Back)* Sorry, but I cannot control them. *(Alternative back)* But you exasperate me when you try to control me.

4. *(Front)* It really sucks for family and friends of bipolar patients. *(Back)* Ha! Try bipolar from my side of it.

5. *(Front)* Mania sucks, but… *(Back)* It sure beats depression!

6. BIPOLAR. There, I said it.

7. Bipolar? Me too!

8. Stigma is so nineties!

9. Mental illness is just another chronic disease.

One morning at about 8 a.m., Rob came down to check on me. I had not slept at all yet. I'd made some notes about "Rob & me & bipolar" that I shared with him. My main insight was that we used to be two in our marriage, but now we were three: bipolar had simply moved in and established herself as another partner. Or was it in fact now *four* of us, since it is *bi*polar after all… I wrote:

> Rob, I've loved you so long. You're my rock, my right hand, my life.

He smiled wanly, hugged me, tucked me in like a little child, urged me to get some sleep, and left.

But I *couldn't* sleep just because someone told me to! Less need for sleep is a key symptom of (hypo)mania, after all.

At around noon, still unable to sleep, I finally snapped. Something set me off and I became hysterical, sobbing and totally out of control. This was the eye of the storm. I had to talk to someone, but I didn't want to be seen like that by Rob or the children. So I tried to call my friend Navid, but she was out. Another friend, Leyla, was hosting a big party that night, so I had mercy on her. I did get through to my uncle, Sturla, the psychiatrist in Toronto, and then to my friends Barb and Judith. With each call, I became slightly less distraught. It felt so good to reach out and make contact with people who were not angry with or disappointed in me.

As if I'd been thrown a lifeline.

I'll never again underestimate the healing power of simple human contact and kindness for people with a mental illness.

With hindsight, I now realize that this was probably an episode of "mania with mixed features" (see Appendix 1), since I had the classic signs of mania together with extreme agitation, anxiety, irritability and bursts of tearfulness.

Mania is like a night at the carnival, fireworks and all. Until it turns ugly, that is. Then the irritability and anxiety can overwhelm.

That night, the whole family apart from Rob – who's not a party animal at the best of times, and this was, after all, the worst of times – went to the party at Leyla's house. I'm surprised they let me out of the basement! I was acutely conscious that I needed to be on my best behaviour so as not to upset my family or friends. I was walking on eggshells in case I misbehaved, but Navid assured me that my behaviour was entirely appropriate. I enjoyed the party, and it felt great to be out of my self-imposed dungeon cell for a while.

At the same time, by the end of the evening I was exhausted from the mental strain of trying to "pass for normal." It was a comfort to crawl back into my private little den in the basement at the end of it. There, I could relax. No observers, no judgments, no pretense.

Late that night, I had another mental storm, and was too restless and agitated to write the post-its myself, so I called Rob, who kindly played secretary for a while. I don't recall saying this, but the first thing in his handwriting says:

Why don't you read my note?!

Was I referring to the sign outside my door saying "Please knock", perhaps? But then, ominously:

> If I kill myself, will you read my suicide note? Notes
> help to record feelings in the vortex.

I don't remember feeling suicidal that night, but clearly there must have been something going on to prompt that.

In a frenzied flurry, I then dictated a series of eleven technical questions about medications, doses, and side effects for Rob to check with Sturla when next they spoke. I also said I felt that I was putting too much strain on the family and should be hospitalized.

Whaaat? Hospitalized; me? Recall my earlier experiences as a young nurse working in psychiatric wards; the "war stories" I had gathered; my fear of and revulsion with mental illness in general.

And now here I was, willingly suggesting that I be admitted to a psychiatric hospital.

How the mighty have fallen...

Next morning, Rob reported back. Sturla said that they only hospitalize people who are a danger to themselves or to others (i.e. suicidal or homicidal). Rob didn't feel we were there yet. This was enough to reassure me for the time being.

Two days later, we had one of our final sessions with Lucy at Friends for Mental Health. She was moving to Ottawa and had suggested that we have a session of art therapy with the whole family before she left.

The session went smoothly, although we were all initially a bit on edge about the "family" and the "art" and the "therapy" parts of "family art therapy"!

The exercise involved each of us first drawing or painting something to symbolize how we were feeling about our place in the family at the time. Then, when we were ready, we pinned our individual drawings on a board, taking into account where others had placed their artwork. For example, one child clearly communicated their feelings of isolation and distance by pinning their drawing in a corner, far from all the other members of the family…

I don't recall this, but Tami tells me I didn't want anyone to place their artwork anywhere near to mine: I was off in my own mad bubble, with no space for connection to, awareness of, or distraction by others.

My drawing from that day shows a terrifyingly giant wave with mean red spikes going all the way up and down. The wave represents a (hypo)manic episode, and the spikes are the irritable surges and mental storms that occur during an episode. I'm in the centre of this monstrous, jagged wave, wide-eyed, howling and helpless.

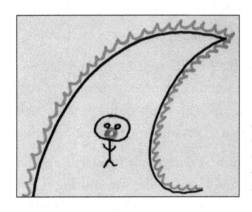

A replica of my art therapy drawing. (I've never had any artistic ability, and this clearly didn't change during mania!)

In many ways, I felt disconnected from my true self while I was manic. It was as if I were looking down on myself from some calm higher plane, observing all the chaos and crisis on the pulsating plane below. I knew the episode would pass, so

I didn't panic too much, and parts of me took perverse pleasure in the antics of manic-me. It was like watching a speeded-up movie of myself.

Some of the things I did were rather odd, such as sneaking out of the house to walk to the lake at 4 a.m. some mornings after no sleep, enjoying every minute of the solitude and making profuse post-it notes about all my insights and observations. Other things were quite uncharacteristic, including spending money much more freely than usual. Even the distressing incidents were strangely satisfying to observe. Like that panic-attack meltdown that left me sobbing uncontrollably and phoning random people in desperation. But the sheer drama of even that commotion swept me along and kept me watching, curious to see what would follow.

And the whole time, while I was keenly aware that my brain was playing cruel tricks on me, I felt powerfully protective of her; fiercely maternal. This precious, delicate organ needs to be defended against naysayers; guarded against those who would judge or scorn her. She's mine, after all, and family sticks together. I felt like a young mother whose two-year-old is having a wild tantrum in a supermarket; she still loves and accepts her child unconditionally and tries valiantly to shield her from critical eyes.

Chapter 7: Mania continues

Speaking of tantrums, at the height of my manic tantrum, Tami pushed for the two of us to get out of the house to take a break. Back in August 2008, when I was just coming down from that first dreadful summer of hypomania, she had started a tradition of us taking one- or two-day retreats at a nearby hotel. We went again in January 2009 when I was stable. For those first two trips, either Karrie and Matt or just Karrie came too. Rob was neither interested nor invited. This time, on June 3, 2009, Karrie and Matt chose not to come: too much madness in too close quarters? Tami seemed unperturbed by being left in charge of me for the night; she intuitively knew how to handle me. In turn, she trusted that I would try not to embarrass her, and I promised to "behave" the whole time.

Promises, promises.

As we entered the ornate hotel lobby, I breathed a deep sigh of contentment. Imagine: nobody here knew I was mad! And if I played my cards right, nobody would find out, either. I stalked self-consciously up to the desk. Am I walking normally? Do I look calm? Am I pulling my rolling suitcase like a sane person would? Check-in went smoothly, and soon Tami and I were settling in to an elegant suite with a magnificent view of the garden and lake. We felt like princesses, and the afternoon, evening and morning ahead stretched out languidly, promising both tranquility and fun.

We started our afternoon lazing on luxurious deck chairs on a dock that extended deep into the lake. Paddle-boats and canoes were tied to the dock but using them seemed too much like hard work. When we'd had enough restful loll-ing, we swam in the indoor pool, soaked in the hot tub, and sweated in the steam room. In the pool, we cavorted like chil-dren, racing each other, splashing, and floating on noodles. Next, we borrowed bicycles from the hotel and rode at a lei-surely pace all the way along the lakeshore to the nearby town. It was exhilarating to cycle, sun and wind against our skin.

Having worked up a good appetite, we showered and dressed for dinner. It was then that I realized my eyes were playing tricks on me. I wasn't exactly hallucinating, but I was having what I called definite "visual effects." It started up-stairs when I had a piece of chewing gum, and the green foil wrapper suddenly looked like shimmering, glimmering emer-alds – the most breathtaking colour I had ever seen. I had bought this brand of gum many times before but had never noticed anything remarkable about the wrappers. Con-cerned, I showed it to Tami to see if she could see what I was seeing. No, it looks normal, she said. (I kept this wrapper with my notes, and as I write now I'm looking at it again. It's shiny, yes, but it doesn't astound me in any way. Strangely, I almost miss that heightened visual sense. But of course it would be unthinkable to wish for the mental instability that caused it in the first place.)

Then, on the way to the hotel restaurant, I looked at the spectacular display of upscale fake flowers on the enor-mous table in the lobby. They beckoned me – emotionally, I mean – to move closer to inspect them. I was overcome with awe and reverence: these were by far the most magnificent flowers – real or fake – I had ever seen, and the colours were astonishing, otherworldly. I felt so privileged to be able to admire them, like someone granted private access to a secret treasury. I was moved to tears and told Tami I had to call Rob to tell him how incredible these flowers were. When I got through to Rob, I was weeping openly, and I tried hard to explain what a special experience I had just had. He must have shaken his head listening to me ranting on about it.

Still on the phone to Rob, I walked slowly down the hallway towards the restaurant, and passed a huge oil painting on the wall. It looked to me like it had been painted by one of the great masters. Again, I was overcome with emotion and wept, saying it was so amazing because the branches on the trees were waving, and the leaves were quivering and dancing.

When I hung up and recovered my composure, Tami and I went into the restaurant for dinner. My hypersensitive eyes immediately isolated what I call a "visual abomination." There was an imposing, round mahogany table near the entrance that had a broken piece on its central leg. Someone had used a large, unstained pine shim to stabilize the table. So you had this magnificent, majestic dark table with a cheap, anemic shim showing. It was a disgrace and I refused to be seated until the manager was called. I angrily explained that the shim was unacceptable and offensive to guests and demanded that a craftsman be engaged to repair the table properly. He politely said: "Yes, ma'am; I'll do my best to get it fixed as soon as possible." I could tell that he found me weird, or worse, mad.

Poor Tami accommodated me through all these dramas, and we eventually shared a delicious meal.

Safely back in our suite after dinner, I decided to listen to some Enya music on iPoddy to soothe me. One track featured the sound of waves. Listening to it, I had my first "auditory effect," like the strange visual effects earlier.

First, the sound of the waves reminded me of my years as a nursing student in Durban, South Africa, on the Indian Ocean. Then I thought of Hawaii, which I have always dreamed of visiting. I also thought of my recent art therapy spiky wave image for mania. Finally, I imagined myself standing on a beach, listening to the waves. No, I was *in* the water, and the waves were breaking over me. No, no. Get this. I *was* an actual wave. I rose, crested, paused expectantly, then released and crashed, furiously frothing and rushing up onto the shore before retreating to the waiting water, leaving a fizzing frill of foam on the saturated sand. As I listened, spellbound, to the music, I was utterly transformed. I *became* those waves. It was uncanny. I lingered there, submerged in that magical ocean-world, rising and falling, being one wave after another.

Then some primal part of my brain sent a cautionary signal. "Maybe it isn't very wise to amuse yourself with your newfound super-senses like this? Next thing, you'll really hallucinate or something."

Reluctantly, responsibly, I removed the earbuds.

How dull: dry land again.

For the evening's entertainment, we watched *Coraline*, an animated film about a girl who travels between the real world where her actual family lives, and a sinister alternative reality where her "other family" lives. I went wild over the fantastic colours and the way the psychedelic tunnel between the real world and the nightmare world seemed to emerge from the TV screen and come towards us, as if it were in 3D. At one point during the movie, I started sobbing hysterically, and when I tried to speak it was total gibberish. Tami was lost: she had no idea what I was trying to say. She was understandably worried, and considered phoning Rob, but decided not to. She didn't want him to get angry with me again. She figured I would soon sleep it off and be a bit calmer in the morning.

Luckily, she was right.

The next morning after breakfast, we went back down to the dock and lounged on the deck chairs until Karrie arrived to fetch us. What a glorious respite it had been. We were both very reluctant to leave and return home.

The hotel supplies small pads of blank notes on the desks in each room. After our short stay, I had filled sixteen notes with ideas. One shows me as a stick figure, running with arms extended behind me, and a heavy, dark cloak falling to the ground, being shed. The caption says: "The cloak represents bipolar." That's how I felt: constrained by an oppressive external object that I needed to cast off so I could run freely again. I loved that image, and I loved that my brain could generate such images for me. Oh yes, I still loved my poor old brain, even though she had lately become so unreliable.

We went directly from the hotel to another spa visit. Karrie and Tami tell me that I was effusively chatty and treated the young woman working there – whom I had never met before – like my best friend.

That night, I went with Karrie, Tami and a friend of Tami's, to a Sarah Slean concert downtown. I had been listening to Sarah virtually non-stop on iPoddy and was really looking forward to her performance. I wasn't competent to drive, so Karrie drove us. I was a nervous wreck throughout the trip. I sat in the back with Tami but was so anxious and jumpy about the traffic and Karrie's driving – which is perfectly safe, by the way – that I grabbed a big, black shopping bag and pulled it over my head and shoulders. I'm serious. With the bag and iPoddy to the rescue, I made it there without having a complete breakdown. It was a close call. I was exquisitely excitable.

The concert was wonderful! The girls say I sang along with great gusto. Worse, they tell me that I was the only audience member singing along at all. They moved to a different part of the hall to avoid me, but kept me within eyeshot, just in case.

Afterwards, I strode over to Sarah's manager and started negotiating for Sarah to accompany me on some mythical "tour" I was planning. Maybe a book tour for this book which at that stage was a mere notion and a clutter of scribbled post-it notes? He was kind enough to humour me politely.

We eventually met Sarah when she came out from backstage. I recall posing for a photo with her and buying all kinds of promotional swag.

Big spender, again.

On the way home I screamed at Karrie about her driving: too fast; too close to the car ahead of us; too slow to brake; whatever. Tami told me later that there was nothing at all wrong with Karrie's driving, and that having me yelling from under my shopping bag while her friend was in the car was really embarrassing.

I dare say.

The next day I scribbled a post-it:

My spiky, prickly brain is calming ++. Rob is really
sick – he has no energy to fight!

Both he and Tami got a terrible dose of the flu and stayed in
bed for several days.

As well as being physically ill, the bipolar steamroller
must surely have flattened them emotionally.

At midnight that night, I emailed Rob:

Hi my beauty,

It's nearly midnight and I just finished eating another AMAZING dinner cooked and frozen by you
last week.

Thank you, thank you, thank you for all that ready-
to-go protein. I really appreciate it.

I love you so, so much.

The following afternoon, Rob dragged himself down from
bed to check emails, and responded:

Hello lovely,

It's such a relief to see you coming back again – from
that whirlwind galaxy we simply have no idea about.
I know we are going to find a cruising altitude that
will sustain you and put you back in the pilot's seat.

Hang in there, my beauty. Love you.

That weekend, I flounced off to the local spa again (by taxi,
as I still didn't feel safe to drive) for a pedicure and a facial.

Wow. Talk about being pampered. And talk about indulgence. I would never normally have splurged for even one of those treats, let alone two in the same session! What is it about (hypo)mania that makes people spend so freely?

That same day, I wrote:

My galloping steeds are now grazing in the pasture. *[Then, in a fit of honesty, I added:]* Well, maybe *trotting…*

As much as I enjoyed the spa, it didn't help me sleep at all. That night I got four hours' sleep spread over three short sessions. I slept from 2 till 3:30 a.m., when I startled awake with heart thumps. I slept again from 5 till 6:30 a.m., when I again woke abruptly, heart pounding. I crept upstairs from the basement to make some breakfast and check emails. I then slept from 8:30 till 9:30 a.m., and was yet again jolted awake.

The next day, Tami and I went back to the spa for yet more pampering. While she had a facial, I had a manicure and back massage. Heavenly! I handed over my credit card without a second thought about the total I was tallying up.

On June 9, Rob drove me to an emergency appointment with Dr. Y who had agreed to see us again in view of my manic symptoms. Rob came both to drive me (I still felt too "racy" to drive safely) and to listen in and ask questions. The appointment lasted over two hours. This was an important date, because – as I explained in Chapter 5 – it was when Dr. Y reviewed my case and changed my diagnosis to Bipolar Type I, rapid cycling (Appendix 1). He wanted to change my medications accordingly, adding either Zyprexa or Epival to the lithium I was already taking. He strongly recommended that I stop taking all the naturopathic remedies I was still on. Also, because I had asked for it, he gave me a referral to the Douglas Institute.

That afternoon, I did research about Bipolar Type I on the Internet. I printed out many pages about the disorder itself, its causes, treatments, and medications. I wasn't really in a state to absorb all this, but I tried. I also made a note to ask my naturopath what the treatment plan would be if I decided to wean off lithium. This shows that even then I was not yet entirely committed to the psychiatric treatment route.

Slow learner?

The following day, I was still in big spender mode. To get out of the house for a while, Tami and I went for a coffee at a local café that also sold second-hand and antique furniture. I immediately spied four elegant oak dining chairs and fell instantly and irrationally in love. To my eye, they were the most handsomely crafted pieces I had ever seen, and I wanted to adopt them without delay. Thank goodness Tami spoke some sense into me, and gently suggested that I phone to consult with Rob before making a purchase like that. Well, I don't need to tell you how that turned out. To this day, I grieve for "my" classic chairs, and wonder if they are well treated wherever they are now.

Five days later, the hurricane had finally weakened. I moved back upstairs and was even able to accompany Rob to a business meeting downtown, where I barely spoke but provided smiles and nods in all the right places. On the way home, we visited the Douglas where we met with Nancy Poirier, one of the psychologists working in the Bipolar Unit. She explained a bit about their mindfulness-based cognitive therapy (MBCT) program. That interested us enormously, as we had read how helpful MBCT can be for bipolar patients.

After the meeting, I asked Rob to drive around the sprawling campus of the Douglas. I wanted to see the distance from the river, the layout of the various facilities, how the different buildings were linked by a network of roads and tunnels, the parking areas, the access to the Emergency Ward, and the inpatient ward that Nancy had mentioned where bipolar patients are usually admitted. Rob humoured me, thinking that it was so typically thorough of me, but surely not necessary. I would never need Emergency! Never need admission to a ward! The worst was behind us now, he believed. I was on effective meds, and it was all smooth sailing from here.

Optimistic, but extremely naïve, as we later discovered.

For me, the self-guided tour of the Douglas helped me feel more secure about switching hospitals. Who knows, maybe I had a premonition about the dramas yet to come. Or maybe I was just being a control freak, as usual. At one point, I went up to Ward CPC2 – the bipolar ward Nancy had mentioned – while Rob waited in the car. I walked, wide-eyed, down the cold concrete corridor, remembering my days as a student and graduate nurse in South Africa. Do they use the same uncaring architects for all these mental hospitals, I wondered? I entered the elevator and rumbled upstairs. At the ward, I peered around to see what I could glean about both the staff and the patients. It was quiet at the time. Things were calm and relaxed. I went to the desk and told the nurse I was going to be a patient at the Douglas and would like to be shown around the ward, please. She stared at me as if I were completely crazy. Well, of course I was, but I still wanted to see the ward, please! "I'd like to know what to expect if I ever have to be hospitalized." She stood her ground and politely escorted me back to the elevator. Seems that guided tours were not provided there! Oh well, nice try. At least I had seen the nurses' station and the dining room/lobby area. Better than nothing, I suppose.

The next day, according to my agenda, was a "Recovery Day." Aah; the end of an era. I went biking, unpacked all the suitcases from my basement room, and even did a bit of work with Rob.

All in all, a good day.

I felt like I had been on an arduous hike through rough terrain and thick bush, and was now emerging from the forest, so grateful to see the light and feel the sun on my skin again. I had been totally lost in those woods and felt scared and alone in there. Now here, at last, were some familiar signposts.

Looking back on this episode which lasted from mid-May to the end of June 2009, I drew myself as a stick figure with my arms extended in pure joy, head thrown back and a huge grin on my face. I'm floating up into the air like a helium balloon. Rob is below me, stretching up to grab my ankle and shouting: "Yikes; you're going up again. Let me hold you down." That's how most of the episode had felt.

Two days later, I drew a big smiley face: "Just so happy to be back!"

Scanning this list of random points from a sample of my post-its will give you some idea of how my brain was firing during this episode. Many other post-its have already been referred to above, so are not included here.

These are in chronological order.

1. How many couples get divorced after one of them develops bipolar?

2. Do people ever die by suicide during a manic episode?

3. Who looks worse these days: Rob or me?

4. Adapt Sarah Slean's song *Please be good to me* for mentally ill people. (Like Elton John adapted *Candle in the Wind* when Lady Di died.)

5. Why did I get bipolar at age 51? Menopause?

6. What are the rates of bipolar in the Third World?

7. Need yoga for mentally ill patients.

8. What have you given up for bipolar? What have you gained?

9. What movies have been made about bipolar?

10. I'm back!

11. Discrimination. Stigma. Shame. Fear.

12. Is bipolar me or an invader of me?

13. Embrace it! (Bipolar.)

14. Name it; say it; own it. "Kiss the scar."

15. "Pass for sane."

16. "SORRY." Sorry I have arthritis/diabetes etc. – if it offends you. (Mental illness is just another form of chronic disease...)

17. Normalize it. "Who in *your* family is mad?"

18. Rob needs a support network.

19. Rob is at breaking point.

20. Mania feels like a volcano erupting in my brain.

21. Check YouTube for images of erupting volcano & giant waves crashing.

22. Research criminal cases involving madness.

23. Watch *Beautiful Mind* again.

24. I should write a book about all this.

25. "Mad as a hatter," etc. Collect other expressions about madness.

26. Does this mental buzzing, fizzing, "bizzing" (nice word: like "busying") fry my neurons?

27. Develop a series of cartoons to explain what this feels like.

28. How can I "switch off" the light? (The glare is blinding me!) It's like neon, flashing!! If I go into a dark room and lie down, will that calm me? Or a relaxing bath with candles?

29. Now a family history of bipolar is hanging over Karrie, Tami and Matt.

30. Draft a "Bipolar Manifesto" for family, friends, colleagues, casual acquaintances, etc. Intro: I have Bipolar Disorder Type I. This means… Depression… (Hypo)mania. How I feel. What I look like. What I need/want from you to help. What I don't need. What I won't want to do but must (e.g. exercise). What I will want to do but mustn't (e.g. spending spree, stay up all night). Good to remember: I love you just the way you are.

31. Songs: "I love you just the way you are." Yeah, right! "Slow down, you move too fast… feeling groovy." "Bridge over troubled water: When you're down and out…"

32. Do you think I'm crazy? You drive me crazy.

33. Need a "divorce prevention plan."

34. 5 a.m.: Gone for a walk. I'm fine but I can't sleep! 6:15 a.m.: I'm back. Goodnight! 8 a.m.: Still no luck sleeping. Will try again now.

35. *[After family art therapy session.]* Rob says: "We have bipolar." Like he used to say: "We're pregnant." He says: "It's a family disease, not an individual one."

36. I see my shadow, so I still exist. I am! A shadow of my former self?

37. The light is not on in depression.

38. Can I focus my thoughts? (Harness all this energy.)

39. How many suicide cases are diagnosed or undiagnosed bipolar? Schizophrenia? Depression?

40. My suicide note: what would I say?

41. Very anxious, jumpy re noises, etc. Twigs, loud movie, Rob's voice.

42. 2:35 a.m.: Hi Tami, please come down and see if I am still awake… I'm worried about you. Love, M

43. Karrie, if I sleep well enough, I will come upstairs for exercises at 8:30 a.m. If I don't appear, please leave me to sleep – need to catch up!

44. TO AVOID CONFLICTS WITH ROB, ASK: DO YOU ABSOLUTELY *HAVE* TO GO UPSTAIRS?

45. Take lunchtime pills!

46. *[Tami was playing secretary; my thoughts were so rapid I couldn't sit still to scribble.]* June 13, 2009. Ideas for book titles: Bonding with bipolar; Bargaining with bipolar; Besting bipolar; Bettering bipolar;

Busting bipolar; Bye-bye bipolar. Chapter titles: Bipolar bruises; Buried by bipolar; Burying bipolar; Battling bipolar; Befriending bipolar.

47. Civil rights. Women's rights. Gay rights. Mental health rights. Mad rights?

~   ~   ~

In September 2011, more than two years after this episode, I took a Creative Journaling class. I wanted to try to explain what (hypo)mania felt like to me. This is what I came up with:

I had been calmly paddling along in my canoe, enjoying the scenery and all the sounds and smells of nature. Naïvely, I had assumed that I could travel like this forever.

Then it dawned on me that the river was speeding up a bit. Oh; this is going to be interesting. Then just ahead, I hit white water, swirling and surging around the canoe. It was thrilling, exhilarating for a while. But then it got too frantic, and I feared for my safety. I could hear the rumble of a looming waterfall all around me, and I felt utterly alone in my fragile little vessel. Who could help me? Who would rescue me? Over the falls I went, in a blind panic. Everything went black, and the roaring of the water threatened to burst my eardrums. When I came to, I was lying, shocked and exposed, alone on the riverbank.

Not for long. I snapped to attention and started exploring my new surroundings, excited. The falls were in the distance behind me, my canoe was gone.

Nevertheless, I felt confident that I would soon extricate myself from this dilemma.

Ah; life is glorious!

This episode gave my family and me a glimmer of what true mania can feel like. It clearly foreshadowed what was to come; what eventually landed me in hospital just a few months later.

Chapter 8: More ups and downs

Sane at last! I got two-and-a-half weeks of blissful stability –
so welcome after all the turmoil of mania. I was able to work
full days, and function normally socially and within the family.

What a treat!

Then on July 5, 2009, the note on my daily chart says:

> Consciously tried to fight a slightly "down" feeling.
> Went to the gym; later did aerobics with Tami in
> the basement. Can regular exercise help to keep the
> depressive wolves away? Appetite is a bit off. Will do
> some meditation before bed.

What triggered this initially subtle mood shift?

One day before, we had attended the wedding of a
young friend of the family. It was a joyful occasion all round,
but something about the hubbub and noisy merriment got to
me. I felt the black veil flapping ominously around my head
and told Rob that I needed to go for a walk in the garden.
Just then the rain began, so I was trapped inside the boister-
ous tent, plastering a fake smile on my anxious face and having to be sociable with all kinds of people I really didn't have
energy for. I just wanted to get out of there. When the rain
stopped I escaped and took a break, but I could feel that the
damage had been done. The veil had definitely reappeared.
Within two days, I plummeted over the cliff once again, and
spent the whole of July and the first part of August back in a
dreadful, despairing depression.

I was so deeply depressed that I didn't write any notes at all during this time. It was all I could do to put a mark on my daily mood chart (Appendix 2) each day to show: I am still way down.

In this state, in mid-July, I was evaluated at the Douglas Institute. The psychiatrist who assessed me, Dr. Suzane Renaud (Dr. R), became my psychiatrist at the Bipolar Unit there. Because of the thick mental fog I was in due to depression, I have hardly any recollection of our first meeting. I do recall one small moment when she asked me if I was taking any medications apart from the lithium prescribed by Dr. Y, and I proudly said: "No, but I *am* taking these." I hauled a heavy bag containing all my naturopathic supplements onto her desk. She looked utterly aghast, and slowly turned each bottle over in her hand, reading the labels and mentally *tsk-tsking* at what she saw as my gullibility – even stupidity. She sternly urged me to stop all supplements and take only my prescribed psychiatric medications. It took a while, but I did eventually comply with this advice.

In early August, we rented a cottage by a lake so the whole family could relax together. Kai was visiting from Botswana again, and Mika came from Toronto to visit with him and us. I was still profoundly depressed when the adventure started, and never once swam in the lake – a bad sign for me.

However, my chart does show a definite lightening of mood during this break, so that by the time we left the lake, I was almost out of the depressive zone.

Was it the vacation that brought me up, or would the depression have ended on its own, regardless?

I have no way of knowing, but I'm guessing that the vacation, with all the good vibes and the whole family relaxing together, really helped.

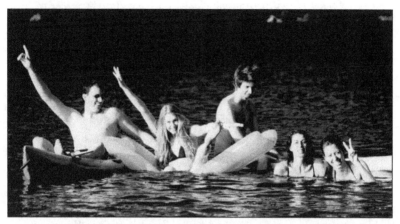

L to R: Kai, Tami, Matt, Mika and Karrie. The five siblings were having fun. Normally, I would have been right in there, splashing and cavorting with them; but I was in depression and merely watched morosely from the shore.

There followed one day – just one day! – of stability.

Next, there was a low-grade hypomania that lasted three weeks. I didn't have to move into the basement, and was able to work quite well, but I was clearly buzzing again and sleeping too little. In fact, this episode was quite interesting. I rated myself on the high side of normal, while Rob rated me mildly hypomanic. But when I look at the notes I kept on the back of my daily chart, it's quite clear that I was unusually elated and energetic. Here's a sample:

> *August 12:* Half a sleeping pill worked for 6.5 hours; couldn't go back to sleep – WIDE awake; ready to get up.

> *August 15:* Great day, but lots of "up" signs: re-decorating and interior design; gardening (uncharacteristic for me); spending money; wanting to socialize

and go out (not hiding in the house); enjoying physical activity; lots of post-its; being a neat freak – vacuuming, tidying, cleaning, doing lots of laundry.

August 16: Worked well. Swam. Great day! Anything seems possible!

August 17: Bad night; only got 3 hours of sleep. Got dreadful news about Gill's [my sister's] cancer and Joyce's [my mom's] stroke on the same day – ouch. But I had no emotion/tears about either – very strange, especially for me. I am somehow divorced from my own emotions these days. Side effect of the meds, or part of the disorder itself?

About two weeks later, on August 30, I went to the gym with Tami, and felt fine. But by the time I drove home, I felt deflated; flat. The dreaded veil came down a bit. After the mini-episode of hypomania, it was time for another two-week depression. The notes on my daily chart say simply:

August 31 – September 15: No energy to write at all.

I did record stints to the gym or exercise sessions with one of the girls in the basement, and those show that despite feeling so flat, I managed to drag my bones out of bed or off the couch, trying to get a rush of endorphins to counteract the depression. I managed some type of exercise on ten of the sixteen days of depression, which I think is rather amazing. No doubt, having a membership at a gym, a personal trainer, and having the kids accompany (drag?) me to the gym helped enormously. Who knows, the depression might have lasted much longer if I hadn't done all that vigorous exercise.

My chart also shows how badly my sleep was affected by the depression. On average, I would sleep for about five hours at night, and then lie awake, ruminating, worrying, and experiencing distressing circular thoughts that bored me because I had been over them so many times before, but I couldn't get them out of my head nonetheless. This anguished mental wrestling match would go on for two or more hours, and then if I were lucky, I'd doze for another one or two hours. The worst was trying not to wake Rob during the tormented time: I wanted to toss and turn, as if I might banish wretched thoughts by changing which side of my head faced up, but I didn't want to disturb him.

Did I have thoughts of suicide during these gloomy sleepless hours? Absolutely. But I never made a specific plan.

I just longed to be dead.

I also mulled over suicide as a way out of my despair during the many hours I spent lying on the bed or couch during the down daytimes. Often, at last, I would drift off and catch up on some badly needed sleep from the night before. My notes show that I napped two, three or four times a day, usually just fifteen to thirty minutes at a time. Those periods of brief oblivion were by far my favourite times of the entire day. Waking up again was utterly dismal: I had to face the fact that my insides felt tangled and knotted and my brain still had a power failure.

Yet now you want me to get changed, put on my running shoes and drive to the gym to join a class of bouncing, flouncing women doing aerobics or Zumba? It was quite a feat. How dutiful I was; how committed to my eventual recovery.

It was mental and physical agony, and I longed for each gym class to be over so I could crawl back onto the bed or couch, and collapse in a still-miserable heap.

Then one morning in mid-September, I woke up and miraculously felt better. I couldn't believe my good fortune. My notes say:

> Finally was able to work for most of the day. What a relief to be back!

This time, I got three days of stability. That's all. It was time for the mood pendulum to swing once again.

On September 19, while still in a stable mood, Rob, Tami and I took our little dog, Nandi, for a walk in the nearby Arboretum. I loved it, but I don't remember it triggering anything in me. I wrote:

> Great day: gym with Tami; walk in Arboretum with Rob, Tami and Nandi! Cooked ratatouille! But no work. I am just so happy to be back!!

Note the unnecessary exclamation marks: a sure sign that my mood was starting to go up again.

On the next day, things heated up. My need for sleep decreased (some nights, I only got three or four hours; others, five or six hours, even though I was taking a sleeping pill every night); my libido increased; and I wrote:

> Great day but maybe some hypomanic signs and symptoms e.g. driving a bit fast; excessively joyful and optimistic; gregarious; "can-cope-with-any-thing" feeling; only five hours of sleep and not at all tired. Help! Rob rated me hypomanic because he

found me impulsive, having a sense of urgency, spontaneous, a bit dismissive of others, pre-occupied with my own concerns, and driving faster than usual. Quite a litany.

So I was already going up, but then the news came from South Africa the next day that my mom, Joyce, since her stroke last month, was "getting worse fast." My sister, Gill, emailed: "She may not last the week." What a day! But even this awful news didn't stall the hypomania.

There followed a week or so of extremely emotional emails and phone calls about Joyce. I felt totally helpless being so far away. I got updates from various family members and from staff at the seniors' home where my mom was living, but I would have given anything to get on a plane to go and say my farewells to her in person. But I clearly wasn't at all fit for a long trip overseas.

During all this drama, I made a note that:

Rob is being rude, snippy, sarcastic, judgmental and abrupt with me. It happens every time I go up; never when I go down. He drives me crazy.

Oh; crazy, eh?

Just as this two-week episode was coming to an end, on October 2, I had my first follow-up appointment at the Bipolar Unit at the Douglas with Dr. R. Rob came with me. My notes say:

Dr. R said that based on my history, I have always been "hyperthymic" (exceptionally high energy, outgoing, happy, productive, etc.), over-achieving, and a perfectionist. Now, with bipolar, I will have to tone it down and live a more normal life – a "boring" life, even. Otherwise I will keep having major bipolar episodes of depression and mania. Now, it has to be early to bed, no all-nighters to finish big projects, etc. Pull back from work and social commitments so I can rest and relax; do regular meditation and exercise; eat balanced meals; and so on. She also said I seem to get emotionally over-involved in issues, and that's dangerous for me.

Hmm… make that *over*-emotionally over-involved!

So true.

To try to control the rapid cycling, Dr. R added Seroquel (an atypical antipsychotic) 50XR to the lithium 900mg I was already on. She also prescribed Zopiclone 7.5mg for insomnia when necessary, and Rivotril (a benzodiazepine) 0.5mg twice a day when necessary. Quite a cocktail. In addition, I was still taking a bunch of the naturopathic supplements – which both Dr. Y and now Dr. R had pressured me to stop – including high doses of vitamins B, C and D, various minerals like selenium, calcium, magnesium, iron, plus thyroid and adrenal extracts, and progesterone. Quite a cocktail, indeed.

The weekend after that first appointment with Dr. R was uneventful, and my mood was stabilizing. But wouldn't you know it, not for long. Three days of stability was all I got before depression struck again.

Starting on October 7 and lasting until November 5, 2009, I was in another draining, dark depression. During this episode I had all the usual signs and symptoms of poor sleep, no appetite, inability to focus, no desire to socialize, no libido, and suicidal thoughts that surfaced and swirled in my wretched mind.

Early in this depression, on October 11, my mom died in South Africa. I had heard details of her slow but steady decline by phone and email. It was awful being so far away. But when I finally got the inevitable phone call to say she had died, I didn't have a tear in me. I felt utterly emotionally neutered, cut off and distant from both the living and the dead. To this day, I have never cried about this loss. Totally uncharacteristic for the pre-bipolar me: I was always really quick to weep, and I had always had a really close relationship with my mom.

Her death has not yet sunk in for me – not at all, actually. Due to the depression and the medications, I was totally emotionally disconnected for the whole month. I couldn't believe how numb and estranged I felt. It was like watching a movie of some other woman getting sad news. I didn't even have energy to make a note about her death on my daily chart.

In mid-October, I started a new medication prescribed by Dr. R, Seroquel 50XR. After a single dose, I slept for 16 hours straight, it knocked me out so badly. When I finally woke and took a bath, I kept dozing off, my head lolling sideways against the tub, drooling with my tongue hanging out. Rob had to stay with me to ensure that I didn't drown.

That's one powerful medication!

A few weeks later, we received a precious parcel from Gill containing some of my mom's favourite strings of pearls and her wedding ring. I held the wrapped parcel tenderly and decided to wait until Rob got home so he could comfort me if I got over-emotional when I opened it. I fully expected to finally crack. When at last I opened it, I gave a small gasp to see and hold the poignantly familiar and cherished items, but still there were no tears. I couldn't believe it: what on earth is wrong with me?

Was it the bipolar or the meds, or maybe a bit of both?

Those four weeks of depression turned out to be the calm before the storm.

All hell was about to break loose.

Chapter 9: Hospital looms

Talk about rapid cycling.

I "switched" out of depression into hypomania over-night, on November 6, 2009. Three days of hypomania later, I hurtled into full-blown mania with psychosis for the first time ever.

If you think mania is a wild ride, try mania with psychosis!

The day I switched, I saw Dr. R for my second follow-up at the bipolar clinic. My notes from that appointment say:

> I told her I have been not only intellectually and socially disconnected, but emotionally, too. For example, I haven't shed a tear for Joyce's death yet; I don't feel bad for Rob and all the stress he is under because of me; I don't relate to the kids – it's as if they are someone else's children! Scary. Awful. I was always so over-involved and over-protective before.

In the margin I scribbled:

> Fighting with Rob all day! Me, irritable and unreasonable; he, impossible and cruel, goading me. I did lots of cleaning and interior design-type. Libido is returning.

Apart from those notes from November 6, I wrote nothing else for the entire month, or for the next few months after that. I disappeared down a mania rabbit hole and was so busy experiencing that otherworldly realm that mundane tasks like taking notes were totally neglected. A mighty manic flood had surged in and swept me out to sea.

I did manage a bit of email correspondence with Mika, who was, as always, wonderfully supportive of me. First, she wrote to recommend some books she thought might help me. I wrote back on November 9 saying I would investigate the books when I was more settled. I added:

> Just pulled a bloody all-nighter despite sleeping pills and the new heavy-duty drug they added to lithium. I give up! But I am singing, smiling, and just SO GLAD to be alive! Which sure beats being in depression, eh?

> Rob was up till 4 a.m. himself, but when he heard me still pottering at 6 a.m., he – on just 2 hours of sleep, remember – got out-of-control angry and picked up the phone, threateningly, to dial 911 to have them take me off to hospital. Total over-reaction on his part, of course, but poor guy. I just smiled gently, and said: "Honey, I'm a nurse and I can assure you, the paramedics will come in here to assess me, and they'll see I'm doing fine, and then I'll ask them to assess YOU, and what do you suppose they'll find?!"

> Ha ha, but it's not really funny...

> Imagine someone with epilepsy is having a huge seizure. Would you scream at her and say: "STOP CONVULSING AND GO TO SLEEP RIGHT NOW, FOR GOD'S SAKE?" Obviously not. You'd wait for the seizure to pass and try to protect her as much as possible while it lasts. Same for bipolar: one of the main diagnostic features of mania and hypomania is "can't sleep/needs little or no sleep" etc. So it's not that I'm being "naughty" or inconsiderate by not sleeping. I'm just being bipolar, Rob!

Oh Miks, I HATE-HATE-HATE depression, but Rob handles it so well. Rob HATES-HATES-HATES (hypo)mania, but I just LOVE it! Well, most of the time, at least.

When all this is over, we're going to need some marriage counselling for sure!

Mika advised me to give Rob some space while I was so wired up. She reminded me that the last time I was manic about six months before, I had moved into the basement, and that had worked well. She ended: "If I were your marriage counsellor, I would say: STAY AWAY FROM EACH OTHER DURING (HYPO)MANIA!"

Wise words, duly noted and obeyed.

Running away from home

I have only vague memories of this incident. Here's what I've pieced together from Tami's and Karrie's accounts.

It was about 8 p.m. and, feeling constrained by my family, I had been trying to escape from the house all evening. So they locked all the doors and kept trying to distract me and escort me back down to the basement where I was by then staying. I waited there just long enough to make them think that I'd given up, then I crept silently upstairs on tippy-toes. Tami does a mime of me looking absolutely ridiculous like the Pink Panther peering left and right, as if sneaking past a security guard or something; she's very funny. But I did eventually fool them and bolted out the front door before Tami could scramble from the dining room to stop me. As I ran jubilantly down the driveway, she yelled for Karrie to come and help and threw on her scarf and coat. Then the two of them dashed down the street after me: Karrie was dressed only in her pink bathrobe and slippers! Luckily there wasn't much snow on the ground yet.

I felt a tremendous sense of freedom and joy running down the street, unrestrained.

When they caught up with me, they tried calmly to persuade me to go back home with them. They each took me by one arm, and gently turned me around. But I somehow unhooked myself from their clutches and sprinted back down the street again. This catch-and-release ritual was repeated several times, and each time I broke free, I yelled: "Help! Help!" They chased after me, shushing: "Shut *up*, Mia! Or the neighbours will call the police!"

At one point, Tami cleverly tried to lasso me in with her scarf. But I ducked. Again, I screamed and sped away, and again they raced after me. By then, I was getting dangerously close to Lakeshore Road with all its bustling buses and other traffic. They urgently needed to get me under control somehow.

Next thing, Rob was there in the car, furious that I had fled from the house. He yelled at me to get in the car. Of course, I adamantly refused. The girls didn't want a scene – or any more of a scene! – so they told him to go back home; they said they'd walk with me to Town Hall and look at some house for sale I said I wanted us to buy. Rob refused to go home, and said he'd meet us at Town Hall, then. He drove at a funereal pace alongside us as we walked, glaring at me menacingly all the way. Or so it felt.

When we got to the house that was for sale near Town Hall, I was all excited, showing the girls how it had a great water view and saying what a good investment it would be. I wanted Rob to see it, and to agree with me. He refused to even look at it. He just dismissed my whole outing as the antics of a madwoman. I was deeply annoyed that he refused to give my brilliant investment idea serious consideration. (In fairness to me, that property was soon sold, the dilapidated old house was demolished, and a beautiful new house with great water views was built. See: it *could* have been a very wise investment. Ha.)

Rob again insisted that I get in the car. I stubbornly refused. We were yelling at each other, which upset and embarrassed the girls. They again told Rob to drive home, and said they would walk me home instead. I was calmer and more cooperative on the way home. At least I'd stopped bolting away from the girls.

They handled me exceptionally well that night.

Rob drove slowly next to us all the way home, giving off what seemed to me to be an aggressive vibe, not a protective one, really. He was hawk-like, not trusting me to make adult decisions. Of course, looking back, I see how grateful I should be that he (and the girls, of course) took such good care of me when I was far from competent to take care of myself. But it did chafe at the time.

It amazes me now to hear about the frequency and ferocity of my fights with Rob in those days. I recall only mild annoyance with him that night. Certainly no yelling. That's just not our style. We've been together for over thirty years, with barely a difference of opinion, let alone a disagreement, between us. But from what the children tell me, when mania entered the mix we both lost all dignity and self-control. Surely such uncharacteristic behaviour takes a toll on a marriage?

Rob says I just became impossibly cantankerous when I went up. He got exasperated and was chronically over-worked and exhausted on top of that. He couldn't wait for me to fall asleep, but even then, he'd never know if I'd wake up and try to run away again. He was always anxious and uncertain. All he could think was: "When will this end?"

Next day, there was another late-late night (well, let's be honest and say early-early morning) jaunt I took down the street in the opposite direction from Town Hall. I had not yet slept at all that night and believed that a brisk walk would settle me. I somehow managed to sneak out of the house un-noticed while everyone slept. This meant first disarming the house alarm, but my exhausted-by-mania family must not have heard the high-pitched *pip-pip-pip* sound as I entered the alarm code. Taking my trusty manic-looking walking stick – a wooden stick that I had liberally decorated with colourful fake flowers, and which I brandished eccentrically on my manic-walks whenever I remembered to take it – I crept out into the still-black, wintery morning, feeling delightfully light and free. No one was about; I had the whole neighbourhood to myself. No one to scold, judge, restrain or control me. It was invigorating to be outdoors, all alone.

I walked a short distance and was suddenly overcome with inexplicable exhaustion. The idea of walking all the way back home was out of the question. I impetuously decided to call Rob to come and fetch me in the car. But I hadn't thought to bring my cell phone with me. Luckily, there was an old age home nearby. Even though it was still an ungodly hour – maybe 4 or 5 a.m. – I saw a few lights on, so knocked to ask if I could please use their phone.

The night nurse looked cautious and concerned when she saw me, wearing a winter coat with sandals and clutching my crazy walking stick, but she kindly let me in. Using all my resources to try to appear sane, I explained that I had been out for an early morning stroll when I had become over-whelmingly tired. She nodded sympathetically, no doubt thinking: "This one's a real nut case."

T-ring, t-ring. T-ring, t-ring... The phone rang many times before Rob's thick-tongued, sleep-filled voice answered, in-stinctively suspicious and anxious. Trying to sound perky and as if I made this kind of call at this hour of the night quite routinely, I told him where I was and asked if he could kindly come and fetch me by car. There was a stunned silence: he could not believe his ears. Now that he was awake, he asked me to repeat my request. I did so, half-wondering if he was just trying to make me feel ridiculous, or if he genuinely had not caught the directions first time around. I could almost feel the fumes from him coming down the wire to scald me. He was completely exhausted from many nights of lack of sleep and had finally been in a deep sleep when I had rudely jolted him awake. Now he had to get dressed and come out in the cold to find me, wandering in the suburban wilderness like the madwoman I was.

I waited quietly, contritely well-behaved, keeping warm inside the old age home. Soon enough, Rob's tires crunched angrily on the snowy driveway and skidded to a halt. He was driving way too fast, that was clear. He *slammed* his car door. Oh-oh. I thanked the nurse profusely for the use of her phone, and resolutely went outside to take my punishment. Rob strode forward, gripped me too-firmly by the arm – as if he were scared I might bolt off again – and frog-marched me to the car. He yanked open the passenger door and shoved me down onto the seat. As if to say: "There. Now don't even *think* about moving." He leaned over and firmly clicked my seat-belt, not trusting me to do that for myself. He then banged my door closed, reiterating his disdain.

As you can imagine, I did not at all appreciate being manhandled. The short ride home passed in stony silence. Chalk up yet another wedge between us.

When we got home, he almost shoved me into the house. I glared at him in bemusement. Why so angry, Rob? I just went out for a little walk, that's all. What harm was done?

Of course, now I realize that a lot of harm might have been done. I might have gotten lost; been assaulted; been run over; wandered onto the lake and fallen through the still-thin ice…

Rob was perfectly right to worry.

Visual hallucinations

I have mentioned the "visual effects" I had at the hotel a few months earlier in the spring of 2009: the green gum wrapper that looked iridescent; the fake flowers that moved me to tears with their beauty; the broken table leg that so irrationally offended me. But those were not real hallucinations.

Though there was that moment in the hotel hallway when the branches and leaves on a painting seemed to move in the breeze. Perhaps that was my first true hallucination?

In any event, on November 9 and 10, 2009, I experienced visual hallucinations that left no doubt. I remember them vividly. Whether they were caused by the mania or were a side effect of Epival – which I had started taking just three days before – I'll never know.

On November 9, I was flying high. At around midnight, wanting to take a break from my over-solicitous family, I went outside and sat on the frigid front porch. I was just scanning the wintery garden, minding my own business, when suddenly a swarm of tiny black dots – not quite flying insects, but something along those lines – came whizzing straight towards me from the pond nearby. As they came closer, I waved my hands in front of my face to shoo them away. But they kept right on coming, flew straight through my hands and head and through the front door behind me. I spun around to watch them go, and then turned back to see if more were coming. Were they ever! Wave after wave of them, all heading straight for my head. It was uncanny. But it wasn't the least bit scary or gross. I was confused at first, but then I figured it out.

I get it! So *this* is what a visual hallucination is like! Wow! I beamed, triumphant at this insight.

After a while, the swarms faded and then vanished. They just melted away. How disappointing! I waited, hoping for more of a show, but no luck. Eventually I got bored and went back inside.

I don't remember this, but the family tells me that I was all excited when I entered and told them all about my hallucination.

"*We* weren't at all excited," Rob wryly notes.

A few hours later, at 4 a.m. on the morning of my birthday, November 10, I was found writhing and groaning loudly on the dining room carpet. The house was completely dark, yet somehow I had managed to creep out of the bedroom without waking Rob and got downstairs without falling in the pitch dark. Then I crawled into a corner, half under the dining room table and between the dining chair legs, where I moaned loudly. Tami remembers incorporating my cries into her dream for a while, but she eventually woke up. When she got to me, she didn't know if I was awake but confused, or whimpering in my sleep. She shook my shoulder and called my name, and I grunted incoherently. Then I mumbled: "What's happening?" She explained that I was downstairs on the floor, and that we needed to get me back up to bed. I was too wobbly from the powerful meds to walk on my own, so Rob – who had by then woken up and come downstairs, too – and Tami supported me to the foot of the stairs, and from there I apparently crawled up on all fours.

I have no recollection of any of this. I had taken one-and-a-half sleeping pills to try to knock myself out for the night, so that probably explains my amnesia.

Not to mention my bizarre behaviour and inability to walk.

On the next day, my birthday, the mania worsened: I was sitting on a powder keg. My manic brain was like an over-dressed Christmas tree, all lit up in blinking, twinkling, glaring fluorescent colours.

We didn't know it then, but I was just six days off being hospitalized.

Again, in the evening, I went out to the front porch. I distinctly remember thinking: "I wonder if the flying dots will visit me again tonight?"

They didn't, but I did experience a much more dramatic visual hallucination.

As I gazed into the garden, hoping to see my flying dots, I glimpsed hints of wispy, colourful steam rising from all the trees. At first it was subtle, but as my eyes adjusted to the dark it became unmistakable. I was initially alarmed: are all the trees on fire? But soon I realized it was just another magical hallucination and I relaxed into the experience.

It was exquisite.

You see, each species of tree emitted its own unique colours – like an aura – and the steamy smoke was whirling in different patterns and at different speeds. For example, the emanations from deciduous trees had much more dynamism, with fast-moving, neon colours; evergreens were more sedate about the whole business. And the steam from young trees positively pranced with power, while older trees were more dignified. The whole yard and the park beyond were transformed into a psychedelic, swirling union of energies. I felt I was watching a 3D movie of van Gogh's *Starry Night* painting. It was entrancing to have a front row seat for this dazzling natural extravaganza.

I longed to get up and twirl among the swirling colours, but that would have been too crazy, even for me. So I remained seated, responsible, mature, well-behaved. Outwardly calm.

But inwardly whirling!

I stayed transfixed for as long as the spectacle lasted, willing it not to fade. I tried not to blink in case the mirage might melt away in that instant. I was convinced that I was seeing the true energy of the trees that was there all the time but concealed from my eyes except when I was in this exalted, altered state of consciousness.

The universe had given me the most precious birthday gift ever.

I'll never forget it.

Mania heightens

After these incidents of running away and the hallucinations between November 9 and 11, my mood chart shows that with each passing day, the mania got worse and worse. As with my previous (hypo)manic episodes, Rob's ratings of me were considerably higher than my own, but even so, it was undeniable – even to me in that state – that we were in deep trouble. Something had shifted with this episode, and I realized, at some fundamental level, that I was not coping on my own.

We were not coping.

It felt like there were runaway, rogue neurons, refusing to be contained within my skull. They poked out of my eyes, causing eerie visual effects; my ears, causing unusual auditory effects; and my mouth, causing me to say cruel things I would never normally have said. I needed to rein in those neurons and get my brain back under control.

But how?

We were all at a loss.

In desperation, Karrie called Mika in Toronto and asked her to come to Montreal to help out. Mika dropped everything and came on November 11. We fetched her from the train station, and after a quick meal together, she and I took a taxi to the Emergency Department at the Douglas.

Fully expecting me to be admitted, Rob had packed an overnight bag for me.

Part 3:

Buried by bipolar

Chapter 10: Emergency visit

My overnight bag was the cause of extreme consternation when we arrived at Emergency and the security guard – an innocent and unsuspecting young man – insisted on searching my bag on the corridor floor in full view of any gawkers and passersby. All my underwear, socks, nightgown and what-not were immodestly displayed for all to gape at. I was mortified at the indignity, and demanded: "Why on earth can't you take me into your office and do the search there, in private?" Mika intervened to get the search over with as soon as possible before I got any more distressed. She knew only too well how prudish I am at the best of times, and she also knew from hard experience over the previous many months that my current emotional reactions were both disproportionate and beyond my control.

On our way into the waiting room, I noticed a large coffee and hot chocolate machine in one corner of the corridor. How sweet! Just knowing it was there made me feel really well cared for. My spat with the security guard just moments before was already long forgotten.

In the waiting room, I befriended a sweet young couple sitting opposite us. After a wait, the woman – girl, really – was called in to see the psychiatrist on call. Mika and I sat quietly, mainly behaving ourselves. I remember being a bit scathing about the suggestion box mounted on the wall nearby: it had neither paper nor pencils available for people to write with. "They must really value our feedback, eh?"

Soon enough, I was assessed by a nurse, and told to wait for the psychiatrist.

During the wait, I went outside for a break. Mika followed and found me guiltily puffing on a cigarette butt. I have no recollection of where I found the butt, or who lit it for me. I hadn't smoked for over twenty years, so this was most uncharacteristic.

When my young friend came out of the psychiatrist's office, she was clearly upset. She took one look at her boyfriend and let out a soul-stirring shriek. She then rushed into the adjacent washroom, where she screamed and sobbed inconsolably. Her anguish echoed eerily off the bathroom walls, magnifying with each gasping breath, and pierced directly into my already severely disordered nervous system. The combination was toxic.

I exploded. Call it empathy. Call it maternal instinct. Call it madness. I don't care. Something had happened to deeply distress my new friend, and I couldn't bear to hear her so distraught. I leapt out of my chair and stormed up and down, waving my arms, and howling and screeching as if suffering intolerable physical pain. "What did he *say* to her? *Why* is she so upset?"

Mika was understandably shocked by my over-reaction, and bravely came over to try to console me. She backed me gently into a corner, where I clutched at her as I collapsed slowly to the floor, sobbing hysterically about injustice and a lack of compassion on the part of the psychiatrist, and shouting over and over again: "But what did he *say* to her? *Why* is she so upset?"

By this time, the offending psychiatrist had peered out of his office to see what all the screaming – in stereo from the young girl and myself – was about, and a group of nurses and other staff emerged from the ward to try to calm us both down.

Despite my torment, I quickly realized I was outnumbered, and also that I was in a position of extreme vulnerability and powerlessness here. So when the nurses helped me up from the floor and firmly walked me towards the confinement room, I relented and went compliantly.

In there, I soon regained my equilibrium, and in fact felt quite embarrassed about the scene I had caused. It had simply been one of those massive spikes on the tsunami of this mania, and it ended almost as quickly as it began. Like a toxic abscess that resolves once the pus drains.

After about fifteen minutes alone, I was assessed to be calm enough to leave.

The staff escorted me directly to the psychiatrist's office. I sweetly apologized for my tantrum, and "played sane" with all the cards in my deck.

I must have put on a convincing show because I wasn't admitted – yet.

I have no further recollections of the evening. I'm told that we called Rob to come and fetch us. Poor him: he had been hoping for a break. I also have almost no memories of the days following this.

It seems the chaos continued.

Four days later, Rob made a note:

3 a.m.: She is still awake, trying to go outside. We give her an extra Ativan (total of 5 today); she finally falls asleep at 4:30 a.m.

9:30 a.m.: She is awake already; gets Zyprexa 5mg. She is very uncoordinated and runs into the door-frame, hitting her collarbone. She throws up. I can't remember if she vomits before or after taking her morning lithium and the half Ativan I gave her. I give her a fast-acting sublingual Zyprexa. Finally, she dozes off.

This gives just a small taste of the drama I put people through during the five days between my first trip to the Emergency Ward with Mika, and my eventual admission. It was too much for my already exhausted family to cope with.

I was both manic and psychotic at the time, after all.

Chapter 11: Admission

Five days after my trip to Emergency with Mika, on November 16, 2009, my family called 911 in desperation and I was duly hauled off to the Douglas by ambulance. Strangely, nobody can quite remember what the "last straw" was that finally caused them to call the ambulance.

I certainly can't: I was much too manic.

I was admitted and spent four days in the Emergency Ward, being stabilized on meds and waiting for a bed on a psychiatric ward. My life had come full circle: I was no longer a judgmental, detached nurse working with psychiatric patients I essentially frowned upon, but a scared, vulnerable psychiatric patient, craving validation, respect and approval from the all-powerful staff.

Although I did have serious beefs with some of the staff, I didn't mind being in Emergency at all. Mind you, I was quite "out of it" most of the time, thanks to the raging mania and the potent new medications I was on. In general, I remember it as a pleasant place to be, and the patients were mostly friendly and accepting.

First night

For my first night, I was on a stretcher in the corridor, just inside the main doors and right below a window in the nurses' station. The public telephone was immediately above my pillow. It was like Grand Central Station there. Normally, I would have hated all the noise, the lights, and being so exposed to the world. But – being so doped up – I was perfectly content. Not a care in the world. I was in my own bubble, and none of the turmoil going on around me penetrated.

My notes next morning say:

> What a drama! In the rush to pack me into the ambulance, they sent me without a suitcase. Had to sleep fully clothed. Slept from about 5–7 a.m. Thank God for yoga pants – woke up looking gorgeous!"

Hmm; I see humility was not my strong suit at the time. Not to mention insight!

Private room

When they finally moved me to a room of my own, just across from the nurses' station, it felt like five-star luxury, and I immediately set about creating a real home for myself. I felt elated being in that private, self-contained space. It was a lovely little room with a curtained window overlooking the counter at one end of the dining room. I fantasized that this counter was a desk in my personal "office." It was important for my identity to feel that I still had use for an office, even in this extreme setting.

I made a long list of items I wanted Rob to bring me from home, and apart from some clothing, I asked for colourful fabrics to use as a bedspread and curtain, and large cardboard boxes that would serve as a makeshift cupboard. Two days later, I asked for office supplies: paper clips, pencils, paper, coloured pens, post-its, clipboards. Like an anthropologist studying an exotic tribe, I wanted to make detailed notes about everything I saw. In fact, I felt compelled to do so. Racehorses in the distance, needing to be captured. As well, these familiar supplies made me feel comforted, secure and oddly competent. Sane, even.

Karrie says the nurses got angry with Rob for bringing in so many clipboards and office supplies. They feared I might use them as weapons, and besides, I wasn't supposed to have so much clutter in my room. But I was settling right in. Nesting. Preparing for the long haul. Making myself at home just as I'd done in the basement room at home.

Just my luck. No sooner had I set up a fully functioning office than I was moved out of my private room into a four-bed ward down the corridor. *Hrmph.*

Post-its and notebook

I have several post-its and entries in my notebook that show I was thinking ahead. One, for example, lists the work-related projects I would need to focus on once I was discharged, and another suggests a "Girls' Night Out" for the group of five or six women I regularly socialized with. As well, I noted that we should take the family to a resort in the Laurentian Mountains. A third post-it says I should get a standing order from Dr. R for daily walks in the yard outside, either under staff supervision, or not – whatever they thought appropriate. I was clearly feeling confined, and the thought that even *prisoners* get a daily walk made me feel stigmatized and resentful. This theme of daily walks followed me to the ward I was eventually transferred to, but unfortunately walks were not on the menu there either.

Not surprising, to be fair, given my recent running-down-the-street antics back home.

The staff

I found most of the nurses in Emergency to be distant, superior, self-important and intimidating.

Just as I would have been in their shoes, no doubt.

They gave off an impatient vibe that clearly communicated: "I'm-too-busy-so-don't-bother-me-now." I would sit patiently for ages outside the nurses' station, observing carefully and waiting for precisely the right moment to ask my question or provide what I felt was valid information, only to leave, discouraged, when a suitable moment never arose. I believed that as a nurse myself, my insights might be valuable, and my approach to the staff especially sympathetic. Even worse than my own disappointment was seeing other patients – my new kin – being shooed along or made to feel bad for interrupting and distracting a nurse from "more important" work. The culture of the ward made it normal and acceptable for nurses to make us all feel inferior, incompetent and bothersome.

Not pleasant.

But in fairness, I see from my notes that we had six admissions in one night. I know from experience as a nurse just how time-consuming admissions can be. Especially psychiatric admissions. And night duty is never any fun, even at the best of times. Let alone in a psych emergency ward.

Maybe I should cut them some slack?

The janitor had a particularly cruel streak and liked to lord it over all of us, playing mean power games instead of being compassionate and helpful. I observed him carefully for a while, and soon thought I had him well summed up. I didn't have the guts to confront him directly – I felt way too vulnerable – so I played a mean trick on him myself. There was a garbage can under the sink in the bathroom. This was useful to drop paper towels in if you were inside the bathroom. But if you were outside in the sitting area near the nurses' station, or in the dining area, and you had a Kleenex or paper napkin or gum wrapper to dispose of, you had to hold onto it until the bathroom became vacant – which could take ages because there was a bath in there as well as a toilet. Why on earth there wasn't another garbage can outside the bathroom I never understood. I arbitrarily decreed that the garbage can should be relocated to just *outside* the bathroom door, so that everyone would have easy access to it. Every time the janitor-jerk turned his back or went on break, I would sneak in and drag the garbage can outside. Every time he saw it there, he'd shake his head in bemusement, cluck, and haul it back inside. This charade delighted me, and I must have repeated it at least twenty times before I was transferred out of Emergency.

You make your fun where you can.

Meals

I just loved mealtimes. The food there gave me great comfort. It was delicious! I'm not joking. Actually, the food was great in two ways: physically and emotionally. Physically, it tasted wonderful, arrived hot, and was attractively served. But emotionally – that was the clincher. It's hard to explain just how pampered and loved I felt to have a tray with my name on it arrive in that oversized stainless steel trolley three times a day, every day. Three times a day, someone prepared food for me. For me! What had I done to deserve this special treatment? It just melted me, every time. I felt like a queen. I was so touched that I saved every menu that came with the meals as precious souvenirs. I wanted to treasure them forever. And I thought I might try making some of these "gourmet meals" for my family one day.

New interests

Something uncharacteristic I did was to obsessively clip articles and ads from the newspapers. I kept these clippings, and it still surprises me to see some of the topics that intrigued me while manic. Things that would never normally have caught my eye suddenly became fascinating: Air Canada seat sales, restaurant specials, an article about pregnant women taking drugs, a report about post-vaccine deaths, and a whole section about health and social services in French, a language I can barely read even when I'm in my right mind. It was as if the mania had literally "lit up" new areas of my brain or caused new neuronal connections to form.

My mind became acutely, exquisitely curious, receptive, expansive.

Suggestions

True to form, I made a long list of suggestions to improve life on the Emergency Ward:

> In the bedrooms: need a shelf or table or nightstand for books, magazines, snacks and a change of clothes. Also need a desk or table with a chair.

> In the bathroom: move the paper towel dispenser to the other side.

> In the common areas: place more garbage cans! Need cards, Bingo, chess, etc. to decrease boredom.

> In the smoking room: empty ashtrays regularly!

> Staff should inform patients of ward rules and ex-
> pectations: for example, mealtimes, times the smok-
> ing room opens and closes, telephone hours, times
> we can get possessions from the staff room, etc.

I never communicated these ideas to anyone – no one would
have cared! – but just making the list made me feel competent, useful, and more in control.

Smoking room

The smoking room was where the serious socializing happened, and it only took me two days before I re-started smoking myself, mainly to fit in and feel part of the gang, but also
to break the boredom of life confined to the ward.

You need to know a bit more about my personal history
and my professional work to understand what a significant
step it was for me to start smoking again. As a teenaged student nurse in the 1970s, I had smoked for a few months, but
my boyfriend hated it so much that I soon quit for him. I
smoked again for a few years with Rob, but we quit together
over three decades ago when I was about thirty.

Since then, as part of my work as a public health consultant, I have researched and written books, articles and conference papers about tobacco reduction, become a smoking
counsellor, and for over twenty years, have made a living
helping smokers to quit and non-smokers not to start.

So, imagine how awkward I felt that first day giving
money to a staff member and asking for cigarettes to be
bought for me. A short while later, a pack with my name
scrawled on it in felt-tip marker was unceremoniously handed
to me.

I took it, reverentially, into the smoking room, nervously wondering if I would still remember how to smoke. (I had no memory of the cigarette butt I had already puffed on outside the Emergency Ward a few days before, when Mika had discovered me.) I needn't have worried: it's like riding a bicycle. I lit up and inhaled deeply, enjoying the familiar, comforting sting of smoke permeating my lungs. It was like coming home!

Offering cigarettes to my smoking buddies was a particular pleasure, and I was notably generous in that regard. I never expected or accepted a cigarette from anyone else, feeling that they should conserve their scarce resources. Did this show snobbishness on my part, or just kindness and concern? I felt I could easily afford these precious – though toxic – little treasures, whereas others might not.

Rob and the children were all stunned to discover my new pastime. Matt says one of the most startling things for him was to see me smoking, knowing how many years I had devoted to helping people quit.

Tami reports that one day I sat her down in the dining area and leaned in close to share a secret with her. I hissed: "Cigarettes are power in here. I use them to exercise control. I give them to people I want to influence, to my buddies, and to people who can't afford their own. And I withhold them from people who annoy me, until they change their attitude!"

One afternoon, there was high drama in the smoking room. I was alone in there at the time, waiting for some smoking buddies to arrive. I heard an aggressive voice in the corridor outside and looked through the window into the ward. The confrontation soon escalated to shouting: a newly-admitted male patient was standing near the nurses' station door, threatening violence. As I watched, several staff slowly emerged from the nurses' station and shuffled into a V-formation, effectively surrounding the man who by now had his back to the wall. I supposed this was some special manoeuvre they had been trained to do, to contain and placate potentially violent patients. The head nurse was speaking slowly and calmly to the man, literally talking him down.

I was terrified, being so close to the whole scene, being alone, and being clearly visible through the large windows of the smoking room. I needed to protect myself.

In a flash of sheer adrenaline-inspired brilliance, I leapt up and dragged the heavy couch in front of the door. I then sat on an armchair facing the couch, extended my legs with my feet on the couch, locked my knees, and, using my legs as braces, blocked access to the smoking room.

Wouldn't you know it, when the man had calmed down sufficiently for the staff to let him move away, he headed directly to the smoking room and pushed on the door. He rattled the handle but couldn't enter. When he peered through the window and realized that I had blocked him out, he shook his fist at me and shrugged his shoulders, as if to say: "What on earth?" I gesticulated back and mouthed: "I'm sorry; I was so scared." Thank goodness, he stalked off, accepting defeat.

It took a long time for my heart to stop thudding, but I was proud that I had protected myself so cleverly. Some part of my brain was still firing effectively!

One day, a sweet but simple-minded older man I'll call Peter was in the smoking room, emptying ashtrays into the garbage as he always did. When he was done, he sat down, lit up and puffed happily. In walked a young woman, not unattractive, but no beauty either. Lily – not her real name – was new to the ward, and she too was at the simpler end of the intellectual spectrum. Peter perked right up when she entered. The two of them made silly small talk while the rest of us – maybe three or four others – looked on in quiet amusement. Their innocuous flirtation was a diversion for us. Then, exhaling his smoke thoughtfully, giving the impression that he had given the matter earnest consideration, out of left field, Peter declared: "I bet you've got a real nice pussy, Lily." Lily was not shocked or surprised in the least. Rather, she paused as if to evaluate his statement critically. I could almost hear the cogs in her brain grinding: Do I, or don't I? How would I know, either way? Peter pressed: "Don't you have a lovely pussy, Lily? I'd love to see your pussy…" This was all entirely too much for straitlaced *moi*. I might be mad and all, but there's a limit to what can pass as casual conversation. I blurted: "Peter! This is totally inappropriate. You can't speak to a young woman like that. You should apologize to Lily."

"But why?" he asked innocently. "I'm sure she's got a lovely pussy!"

No one backed me up, and Lily still seemed totally unfazed, so I gave up and huffed out of the room, shaking my head disapprovingly. I was shocked, but part of me was half-smiling internally at the lack of inhibition of both Peter and Lily. They were fellow passengers on this crazy cruise ship we were all on together, and for that reason, they had my full support.

Friends

I made friends remarkably easily in the Emergency, and with all kinds of people – gangster types, young guys, old women, everyone. When manic, I was unusually gregarious. In addition, we all had this curse of mental illness in common, so there was a mutual understanding, an affinity, an empathy on which we could easily build. We read the signs without too much difficulty: So-and-so is looking withdrawn and sullen – she needs to be left alone; So-and-so is wearing regular clothes, not rumpled pyjamas, and is sitting in the dining area – he looks like he's ready to chat.

The notes I kept show that I was endlessly amused by the antics of my fellow ward-mates. I thought that I might write a play or movie script featuring some of them. In fact, on one page of my notebook, I listed the cast in a play tentatively titled: *Even prisoners get a daily walk.*

I have changed their names here.

There were four of us with bipolar: Tina spent hours counseling me – her main message was that I needed to take care of *myself* for a change; Cathy was gay and obese – she said she had gained all the weight from her meds; Margaret confided that she had transitioned from male to female as a teenager; and there was me.

Then there was a good-looking young man we called "Bon Jovi" because he looked and behaved like a rock star; he was psychotic, presumably schizophrenic. Peter (of "lovely pussy" fame) was a much older man who had probably had a lobotomy back when they were popular. He was always cheerful, but had slurred speech, a low voice, and he staggered around in a hospital gown instead of getting dressed. Rick was a young schizophrenic who wanted to train as a sniper. Yikes! Jeff was twenty-ish, and kind to everyone. Mark was a twenty-something geek, very gentle, in complete shock about being admitted – I never discovered what for. He kept trying to contact his parents to find out why they had put him in hospital. It was painful to watch.

Kevin, who was thirty or so, was a complete mommy's-boy. He would introduce himself shyly: "I'm Kevin, Kevin" but it came out as "Kevin-Kevin" as in a double-barreled name. And he would repeat his name(s) obsessively, a hundred times, until the listener gave up and walked away in desperation. After a day or so of this, I called him "Kevin-Kevin" all the time, but neither he nor anyone else even reacted. "My comedic talents are wasted on you folks," I thought. Then he'd get on the phone to his mother and grandmother (he lived with the two of them) and, in his annoyingly high-pitched, nasal voice, say: "Is that you, Mommy-Mommy? Am I going to come home soon, Mommy? Please, Mommy. I love you, Mommy-Mommy." (And then the exact same pleading conversation with Granny-Granny.)

Finally in my in-group, there was Bill, a middle-aged man who disclosed that he was going to be admitted to a drug and alcohol rehab centre way out in the countryside somewhere. He called home to say goodbye to his children and wept achingly after the call. Full of remorse. Then, under the influence of some legal or illegal, prescribed or not-prescribed substance, he slumped into a stupor on a chair by the phone, head thrown back, snoring roundly, thick legs planted like ancient oak stumps. The next time I paced past, his chin had dropped forward and dark drool was pooling on his chest. I looked away, embarrassed for him. Surely he deserved some privacy while he slept it off?

Overall, a great group of buddies.

Visitors

Even though I have clear memories of many of us in Emergency, I cannot recall any visitors there, not even Rob and the children. Fortunately my dear friend, Navid, took the trouble to write about her visit to me on my first day. She later emailed me her impressions. She said when she arrived I was sleeping soundly. I didn't wake at all, so she went to ask a staff member for a piece of paper to leave me a note. When she returned, I woke up, and when I saw her I got all emotional, flustered about my appearance and wanting to look respectable for her. She told me that we chanted some prayers together, and then I wanted to introduce her to all my new friends. When she was leaving, I cunningly contrived to hide behind her to sneak past the security guards. No surprise, that brilliant escape plan failed miserably, and I was summarily escorted back inside, humiliated and crying. Seeing me so helpless and sobbing then made Navid start weeping, too. My, oh my.

Later, I had recovered enough to phone and apologize for upsetting her. Apparently I phoned again that night to apologize once more.

On that same first evening, our daughter Karrie made some notes in my notebook: I was obviously too incapacitated to write myself. The notes read:

November 18, 2009.

Short-term memory erased: couldn't remember Navid's visit; couldn't remember Leyla's visit; couldn't remember doctors' visits.

Rob and Karrie got me moved into a room instead of being left in the corridor.

That's a rather lean list: I obviously ran out of steam… Nevertheless, I'm surprised that I had the foresight to keep notes at all. The old sociologist in me was still stirring at some level.

For Navid's next visit, she brought me homemade waffles with strawberries and custard that I wolfed down gratefully. Yum! She said: "You were like the boss of the ward, talking to everyone and introducing me to all your friends." I have no recollection of any of this, but I can just imagine myself gliding down the corridors, smiling graciously left and right, feeling utterly at ease. I had fun there.

Home away from home.

Rob's impressions

Rob, on the other hand, was utterly appalled by conditions in Emergency.

He says there was a total lack of privacy – there were people around me all the time, some staring in a dazed or not-too-friendly way. I couldn't move two paces without edging past someone slumped in a chair or pacing mindlessly. He found the staff members completely inaccessible: they only emerged from their enclosed "situation room" to give meds or escort visitors in or out.

He tells me that I hated it there at the time and remembers me being completely distraught. He says I just wanted him to get me out: "Hire a lawyer; do whatever you need to do!" But I honestly don't recall feeling that way. Whatever meds they had me on clearly worked their magic.

Rob wrote an email to all our family members in which he expressed his genuine dismay about conditions in Emergency. He told them that it's overcrowded with some awfully sick men and women all crammed into a few rooms and two corridors. He was concerned that I could not leave, not even if he wanted me to be discharged. To get me out, he would have to get a lawyer and bring a case against the hospital. Once there, patients are entirely at the mercy of the institution, and they make it abundantly clear that if you ask for too much, you will not get much compassion. He half-joked: if you were not altogether insane on going in to Psychiatric Emergency, you would doubtless become so before getting out. He said that having seen what the Emergency is like, he was not too optimistic about what the psych ward will have to offer.

Years later, researching for this book, I asked Rob what he remembered about the Emergency Ward. He said there was no one offering care of any kind; the staff members seemed purposely callous, distant and uninvolved. The whole approach seemed to be non-interventionist. He thought they wanted to make me compliant through intimidation. "Maybe that's what they've found they have to do with mad people just to manage them." After the first night sleeping in the corridor, they moved me from one room to another every day or so. Rob figured they do that on purpose, to disorient patients, to keep us off-balance. He says the environment was one of extreme stress. He doesn't think it helped my recovery at all. When he and the kids visited, I was sometimes cowed, sometimes defiant. I ran hot and cold, sometimes being delighted to see them, and needing them to be there, and other times just wanting them to leave, urgently. He recalled that I was happy with the food, and I started smoking either to join the crowd and be accepted or just to have another area to go to – the smoking room – in that confined, crowded space. He felt utterly helpless. He tried to be there as much as possible to be a witness, and to make sure that the staff knew there were family members watching and advocating.

Rob had very little to say on the positive side. All he could think of was that he was grateful that visiting hours were flexible, and the parking was very convenient compared to most major hospitals.

Not much to go on in a family crisis like this.

~   ~   ~

After four days in Emergency, a bed finally became available for me in CPC2, the psychiatric ward where most bipolar patients stay. (This is the same ward I had tried to get a guided tour of many months before.) I packed my belongings and was escorted – via an intricate system of tunnels that connects all the buildings at the Douglas – to the ward on the second floor of a building across campus.

As the ancient, long-suffering elevator doors lurched open, I peered out nervously, not knowing what on earth to expect.

Chapter 12: Ward life

If you're like I was, the idea of being locked up in a "loony bin" was appalling. Images from old movies and books dominate: remember *One flew over the cuckoo's nest?* And I had all those disturbing memories from my psychiatric rotations as a young nurse.

So I was unexpectedly and pleasantly surprised by Ward CPC2. It was spacious and sun-soaked with generous corridors, and I relaxed into it with ease.

I was admitted to both Emergency and CPC2 twice within two months, so my memories of the two admissions have more or less merged. I was so foggy from the prolonged mania and being on so many meds, I barely knew my left hand from my right. For the purposes of telling my story, I won't try too hard to separate things.

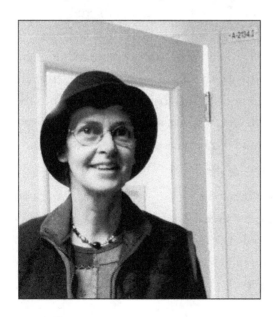

Rob snapped this photo of me in the ward. I wore a hat all day trying to calm myself by having something physical to restrain my racing brain. Even with all the meds, my mania persisted.

My first admission was from November 20 to December 7, 2009, and the second was from January 1 to 9, 2010. So I only had about three weeks back home between the two admissions.

Settling in

My first room was down the corridor and around the corner from the nurses' station, common areas, and the women's washrooms. It had three beds, and I was an "extra" sleeping on a cot on the floor. After a day or so, someone was discharged and I got promoted to a real bed. Now I truly felt I belonged.

What I most loved about this room was the tiny handbasin and mirror. I found it so cute, and thought it was so considerate of the designer to have placed it there for our convenience. I took great pleasure in washing my hands there several times a day, just for the joy of it. (No, don't worry; I didn't have obsessive-compulsive disorder as well…)

Along similar lines, I was thrilled about the fully stocked linen trolley in the corridor near our door. We were free to take whatever linens we needed at any time. Taking clean linen without having to worry about who would eventually launder it was truly delightful. And tossing used linen into the large canvas receptacle with a *th-wump* gave me a strange satisfaction. It reminded me of my days as a student nurse when bed-making was such a major feature of each shift.

Just past our room, at the end of the corridor, were two small armchairs and a coffee table. This sitting area overlooked a beautiful snow-covered meadow and several majestic, mature trees. Immediately, I saw the potential for my next office, and set up shop with my clipboards, notebook, post-its, paper clips and what-not. Nobody seemed to mind that I had commandeered this prime piece of real estate. I felt at peace there, and spent hours in silent reverie, making notes about insights and ideas, many of which have now made their way into this book. Looking back at those notes now, I realize they were quite coherent, all things considered. Some neural pathways were still firing.

Although I thoroughly enjoyed the company of many of my fellow travellers on the ward, having this private little haven to retreat to every now and again provided a break in the daily routine and helped make my stay as pleasant as it was.

At some point I was put in a two-bed room much closer to the washrooms and nursing station. The first few days there were too good to be true: the second bed was unoccupied so I had the room entirely to myself. It was like being in a luxury suite. I had taken the bed by the window, which overlooked the same scenic meadow as my office.

After some time, a new admission was moved into "my room." She spent most of the day facing the wall, sleeping. As soon as she staggered off to shower or watch TV, I made good use of the privacy to do yoga or other exercises: I didn't want to make a complete spectacle of myself in front of her.

Common areas

The common areas consisted of the wide corridors, bathrooms, dining room (my favourite room, because as in Emergency, the food was great), smoking room, small TV lounge, and large exercise room (which had an exercise bike and treadmill, a big TV, and two telephone booths). So there were plenty of places to wander in and out of during the day, looking either for someone to chat to, or a decent TV program to kill time with until the next meal or snack was served.

There were a few highly sought-after rocking chairs dotted around the ward, and I made it a habit to try to get one as often as possible. If a rocking chair were taken when I got there, I would sit as close to it as possible, and leap into it the moment the occupant got up to go to the washroom or smoking room or whatever. It was rather comical, but I found the rocking motion really soothing.

Unlike in Emergency, where we had comfortable couches and armchairs, the smoking room in CPC2 had absolutely no furniture at all. We either sat perched on the frigid windowsill or on the stone-cold floor, or just leaned against the wall, standing. Did they fear that we'd set the place on fire? Maybe the staff didn't want to encourage us to stay in the densely smoky room for longer than was necessary to smoke one cigarette at a time. Nevertheless, as in Emergency, it was *the* place to socialize. In my case, the actual smoking was of secondary concern; rather, I wanted a chance to bond with my buddies. Offering cigarettes to my friends was still a source of great pleasure. (Luckily, I managed to quit smoking without too much effort a few weeks after discharge.)

Telephone calls

I used the telephone an awful lot during my first few days on the ward. I guess it was a link with the outside world, and using it made me feel a bit normal. From my notes, I see that I called the CLSC (local community health centre) and left messages for the social worker there. I also tried to get through to various community organizations, looking for resources and support. It was often difficult to reach people, and if they called me back when I was out of the room, I had to rely on whichever patient answered the phone to come and call me from wherever I was. Of course, many calls got dropped in the process. Regardless, this is how I spent much of my time in the early days.

I also called Rob and the children from time to time, usually to ask for clothing or other supplies to be brought in next time they visited. But I was still quite stung about how they had all treated me while I was still at home (restraining, controlling, and patronizing me), so I was probably secretly punishing them by not calling as often as I might, or not speaking for as long as I normally would have.

As well, I found it difficult to focus and maintain interest in what people were saying – especially over the phone. My head simply wasn't working well at all.

Understatement!

Occasionally, when I felt clear-headed enough, I would call friends as well, but I found social calls to be particularly draining. Which role should I play? Must I try to act normal and cheerful, or could I let my guard down and tell people how overwhelmed and confused I felt as an inpatient in a mental hospital? It was all too much to figure out: social isolation was easier and seemed far preferable.

The staff

Right at the beginning of my stay in CPC2, I wrote:

> The nurses are way nicer over here than in Emergency. Is it just due to their physical accessibility (architectural layout of the nurses' station, behind a

counter here rather than in a fully enclosed room in Emergency), or are they in fact kinder, gentler, more concerned?

Looking back, I would now add: "And way less stressed." By the time patients are sent over from Emergency to the ward, the meds have kicked in and we are generally much more stable; easier to manage…

A few of the staff were excellent: I remember with great fondness two nurses – Nathalie and Robert – both of whom treated me with genuine respect; some were so-so; and some were patronizing, slack or downright mean. I scribbled a note:

> No real nursing care here. They nurse our files, not us! How can they write reports about us if they never leave their 'boat' (staff room) to wet their feet with us? Are snippets and hearsay enough to make accurate nursing assessments? Come out from behind the desk! Especially when a patient is getting belligerent or upset. Beyond the mechanical, "How are you today?", we each need a daily interview or focused interaction.
>
> The nurses don't facilitate any therapeutic – or even social – interactions between us as patients.

In fairness to the staff, as a nurse myself I must admit that constantly interacting with needy, anxious patients and their families – regardless of the diagnoses concerned – can be totally exhausting. In this case, our off-kilter demands and bizarre behaviours must only have heightened their resistance to spending more time with us. Small wonder they stayed behind the counter and chatted among themselves as much as possible.

Night staff members were often crabby and bossy, and that never sat well with me. One night, early in my stay, I couldn't fall asleep, so I decided to sneak past the nurses' station to watch TV in the lounge down the far end of the ward. I figured I'd be safe there, as the nurses should have no reason to patrol – all the bedrooms were on the opposite end of the ward. Heart thudding with excitement at this bold plan, I tiptoed to the bedroom door, peered cautiously left and right to check for any prowling staff, then dropped to my hands and knees and started *crawling* down the long corridor, so I'd be below the level of the counter where the nurses sat. Ha. Just my luck, one of the meanest nurse aides came out and caught me in the act. I felt ridiculous, down on all fours – like a naughty toddler, busted by an angry parent. She glared at me in disbelief, then shooed me unceremoniously back to my room, and gave me a long, hissed lecture about how important it was for me to get good sleep (I had to agree, but don't you get it? I simply *couldn't* sleep), and not to disturb the other patients, and blah-blah-blah. I sucked it up but then rolled my eyes dramatically, like a teenager, as she left. Furious and humiliated, I tossed for hours, longing for dawn so I could walk around without censure.

One morning, I went down to the lounge at 5:30 a.m. and stretched out on the couch with the TV on. There was no one else awake yet. This same staff member strode past to get something from the storeroom nearby and was outraged to see me lying on the couch. "Sit up! The couch is for two people, not one. You can't lie on it like that." As if there were a line-up of people waiting to share the couch at this ungodly hour! Again, I complied, but sighed, rolled my eyes and gave her the finger the moment she turned her back. Then, as soon as her footsteps retreated, I lay back and stretched out in a luxurious and exaggerated pose, thoroughly enjoying this quiet little rebellion.

A night nurse stalked past me as I sat in a rocking chair early one morning. "Good morning," I said, smiling timidly, trying to be friendly. She glanced over at me, as if confused, and kept going without any acknowledgment whatsoever. My hesitant greeting hung in the air, rebuffed, wasted.

At the end of one night shift, I wrote:

> These nurses resent any contact with me – as if I'm a leper! When one took my temperature and weighed me early this morning, she was so grudging about having to deal with me! Treated me like an object. *Hrmph.*

But I must emphasize that negative interactions with the nursing staff in CPC2 were not common. For the most part, things proceeded smoothly in neutral mode, or went really well in the case of the few excellent staff members who did show caring and compassion; who treated me like a woman – a human being – who just happened to be sick at the time.

Occupational therapy

There was a sweet young occupational therapist (OT) who arranged for us to go swimming in the indoor pool, or to pet animals in the zoo-therapy room once a week. I enjoyed both these activities, but felt it wasn't nearly enough activity to get us through the long week. As well, the OT never engaged any of us in therapeutic conversations. In all my time there, I never had a personal interaction with her beyond: "Do you have your swimsuit with you?"

That was the extent of our occupational therapy.

In the exercise room, there were shelves full of blunt, chewed crayons and yellowing, dog-eared children's colouring books, but I hardly ever saw anyone using these pathetic and archaic art supplies.

I made notes to myself suggesting activities like daily exercise (even a simple supervised walk round the outside of the building would have been better than nothing); a daily cultural, arts or crafts activity; an activity to promote reading (e.g. a book club, or magazine article club); and yoga, meditation, aerobics or Zumba sessions to relieve stress. And what about a weekly group therapy or psycho-education session to encourage socialization and development of insight into our mental health problems? We had so much time on our hands, it was a real shame not to put some of it to good use. I wanted to talk to the OT about my concerns, but never got up the nerve. I felt too vulnerable to rock any boats by making suggestions. That would make my criticism of the existing services explicit and might put staff on the defensive.

I'm sure she had other wards to take care of as well, but I often saw her in the nurses' station, just chatting light-heartedly. I figured that she was probably more comfortable in there, with them, than out here, with us.

Psychiatrists

There was a really funny incident with one of the psychiatrists in the ward. Rob and I were in a meeting with him and a nurse, discussing something about my case. The psychiatrist wasn't quite comfortable at the table so he used a lever to adjust the height of his chair. But he pressed the lever while his full weight was still on the seat, so the chair plunged down to its lowest setting. Seeing him plummet down and almost disappear below the table was hilarious, but no one burst out laughing, out of respect. Rob paused, but couldn't resist a wry remark: "Oops; the shrink shrank!" Then we all laughed!

The psychiatrist who cared for me most of the time on the ward was Dr. Wolf (Dr. W), a gentle soul who made me feel secure and trusting from the outset. I only remember seeing him in two meetings with Rob in the ward's conference room, where he explained the changes in medications and where we negotiated for weekend passes from the hospital, and so on. He may well have looked in on me briefly while I was in my bedroom or in one of the common areas, but I don't remember that. Probably he relied on the nurses' reports to know if the medications were working or needed to be changed.

On Friday November 27, Rob and I met with Dr. W and a young medical student to discuss progress. Rob had made a series of notes on a piece of paper: "Immediate objectives? Intermediate objectives? Role of bipolar team and outpatient psychiatrist? Specific issues for rapid cycling bipolar." They discussed all this at length. I sat quietly, on my best behaviour, as their words swirled above my head pleasantly. I was much too woolly-headed to reach up and bring them down into my brain. And even if I had managed, my brain was too spongy to have made any sense of it all. Those are powerful meds they give you.

Rob's notes indicate that Dr. W was putting me on a larger dose of lithium (from 900 to 1,200mg per day), Epival (an anti-convulsant that acts as a mood stabilizer), and

Zyprexa to control mania. The good news I did manage to integrate was that I could have a half-hour pass to go outside into the grounds with a chaperone sometime that weekend. Suddenly I realized how confining the ward really was. Rob agreed to come the next day so he could be with a staff member (it was my favourite male nurse, Robert, who took us out) and me for the big outing. Half an hour of freedom! *Woo-hoo!* No, let's remove those exclamation marks: mustn't get too excited or I might get more manic. Half an hour of freedom. Woo-hoo.

Dr. W ordered a brain scan to "rule out an organic cause for psychosis and amnesia." I remember lying there during the scan, half wishing they would find a tumour which could "simply" be surgically removed, and then I'd be back to normal. At that stage, in that state, a brain tumour honestly seemed preferable to bipolar disorder.

The scan was all clear. I was stuck with my diagnosis.

Visitors

Rob and the children visited daily, and I was usually well pleased to see them. We were all on our best behaviour and they didn't stress me too much.

Rob provided a superior fetch-and-carry service, trundling clean clothes in and dirty laundry out, and bringing clipboards, fresh fruit, snack bars, and other treats. Sometimes I had requests for different clothes, or fabric to decorate my bed and bedroom. He took time to locate exactly what I had asked for. He later reflected: "Some of your requests were a bit strange because you were still a bit manic but being in such a foreign place you needed familiar things to make you feel at home. Often you didn't use what we brought, and we took them back the next day, replacing them with something new."

The kids occasionally – at my insistent requests – played guitar and sang for some of my newfound friends, one of whom played guitar himself. These were wonderful interludes, and we all felt cheered by the camaraderie of the moment. The whole ward warmed up for a while.

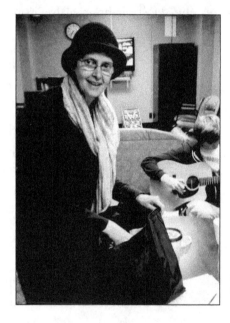

Digging in the bag Rob has brought with my latest requests. Matt, in the background, prepares for a guitar concert in the ward.

Rob always grilled me about any changes in the medications, what the doctor had said, what the treatment plan was. I honestly didn't care about any of that stuff. I was completely docile and passive in the hands of the staff – most unlike me – blindly trusting that they would do what was needed to get me back home when the time was right.

For now, I was in no hurry to be discharged.

My hands were impossibly shaky from the high doses of lithium I was on, so one day I asked Rob to scribble some notes for me:

November 21, 2009.

Only now that I *have* bipolar can I appreciate that there are normal human beings inside the façade of madness. That person is residing there, locked in. I have had to sacrifice so many days, weeks, months to this disorder. In…

The note ends tantalizingly just like that; one of countless incomplete thoughts from those chaotic days.

I never stopped to wonder what it must be like for my poor family to visit me there. Later, they all commented on the unwelcoming approach to the ward when they entered from the parking lot. Dark, cold, grey basement corridors led to the elevator. To them, it felt like a prison, a place of punishment. And when the elevator doors opened onto the ward, the staff seemed to regard them as impostors, not people they wanted to help. But as Rob said, it must be extremely onerous work, managing so many people who are in turmoil, or confused, or not wanting to be there.

Once there, my family found that I was more concerned with introducing them to my latest friends, or showing them off to everyone, rather than actually connecting with them in any meaningful way. My social skills were shot, and my emotions all but shut down. I also felt mortified that I had been unable to avoid being hospitalized. I should have been able to take better care of myself…

One day, my friend Mitra, a naturopath, and her friend, Kim, a naturopath who had been treating me for many months, arrived for a visit. I had no idea they were coming and got all flustered about how I would possibly entertain them on the ward. (Entertainment was surely the last thing they expected from me.) Maybe I was also embarrassed and ashamed to be seen in the hospital? Then, just as my anxiety mounted, one of the patients who had periodic shrieking fits (I referred to her as "The Screamer") let fly with a series of piercing howls. That was enough for me. I physically turned Mitra and Kim right around – they hadn't even taken off their coats yet – and frog-marched them back to the elevator where I dutifully thanked them for coming and said a no-nonsense goodbye.

They were clearly bemused, but obediently left. I rushed to a window overlooking the parking lot and waited anxiously for them to emerge from the building and tramp through the snow to their car. I didn't want to take any chances on getting another surprise visit from them. Fortunately, they got in the car and drove off. I watched like an anxious child until their taillights disappeared behind a neighbouring building, just to be sure I was safe.

Ward mates

The Screamer was moved up to the third floor not long after this, and we would hear her distressing yowls through our ceiling every now and then. "Better them than us," we'd all think. I never knew what caused her anguish. She was in a wheelchair, but her pain didn't seem to be physical; it was deeply psychic, in my opinion.

Apart from The Screamer, there were several other memorable characters on the ward. My best friend was a Haitian voodoo practitioner, palm reader and psychic who gave me a lot of unsolicited counselling on all kinds of matters. She was great fun to spend time with.

There was an older woman who always wore the most outlandish make-up: raccoon-style eyeliner, clownish rouge applied in bold circles too high on her cheeks, and crimson lipstick that strayed way north and south of the edges of her actual lips. She looked like a parody of a drag queen. I wondered if maybe her eyesight was so weak that she couldn't see how hellish she looked in the mirror. Or maybe she didn't bother to use a mirror at all?

One friend, Cathy – who I had met in Emergency – was seriously overweight and confided that she had almost doubled her weight since starting her bipolar meds, gaining 100 pounds in just one year. I shook my head in disbelief: is that even possible, I wondered. Little did I know, before too long it would be my turn to test that hypothesis.

There was a glamorous young woman with social phobia: if she was in the smoking room, she had to leave if more than four of us were there at the same time. She wore the most elegant and avant-garde headscarves: it was like a fashion parade every morning as we all checked to see what she was wearing that day. I don't remember this, but Tami tells me that I asked this woman to teach me how to tie a headscarf. One day, when the family visited, I was swanning around with a spectacular scarlet silk scarf on my head, a loan from Scarf Lady. The tassels hung exotically like long bangs on my forehead. Now that she mentions it, I do vaguely remember flicking my head left and right – in a somewhat provocative way, you understand – to get the "bangs" out of my eyes. I'm told I was immensely pleased with my new look. As well, having a scarf tied tightly like this maybe helped keep my unruly neurons in check?

About a week into my stay, Scarf Lady – normally withdrawn and quite sullen – started glowing radiantly and sported a Mona Lisa smile. It soon became clear what had changed: she was in love. She and one of the male patients – let's call him Lover Boy – had hit it off and were now inseparable. This lasted a few glorious days, and then something must have gone horribly wrong. We woke up one morning and Lover Boy had been "disappeared"; whisked away to another ward in the night. Scarf Lady was inconsolably heartbroken. It was upsetting to watch her pining like that.

The day of Lover Boy's disappearance, we found out that he and Drag Queen had also had a fling – wow! how was *his* eyesight? We never heard whether this had happened before and/or during his romance with Scarf Lady.

Who knew that such a convoluted romantic drama was unfolding right there under our noses?

There was another set of young lovers, both with bipolar, who met on the ward and paired up, but luckily for them were never separated. They were making plans about how they could continue their relationship after discharge.

One day, I overheard a new arrival to the ward – a young Muslim man – sullenly ask the nurse: "Where can I go to pray?" The nurse was flummoxed; she had never had a request like this before. I had a bright idea. I offered the man one of my colourful African cloths to use as a prayer rug on the floor in his bedroom. He gratefully accepted. Potentially awkward interfaith incident averted.

One woman arrived towards the end of my stay and irritated me intensely with her constant gushing chatter during TV shows and movies. "Oh my God, did you see that?" (*Duh;* we're all watching the same thing as you; of course we saw it.) "Ha ha; just look at that, will you?" "I've never seen anything like that in my whole life!" And so on, all the way through. Even relaxing in the rocking chair didn't calm me down. I'd leave, and either go to the smoking room, to my office, or lie down on my bed to escape her. What goes around, they say. Now I knew how my own wretched family must have felt listening to manic-me babble on incessantly.

I was pleased to make a few very good friends on the ward. It felt a bit like boarding school and nurses' residence all over again: we were all living in close quarters, sleeping in dormitories, sharing a large bathroom, eating communally, and constantly looking for things to do to break the boredom but not get us into too much trouble with the authorities. We moved in small packs, and would try to get seats together for meals, decide which TV screen to go and vegetate in front of and when to take a hard-earned trip to the smoking room – the highlight of the hour. We seldom divulged anything personal about our lives-out-there, but when visitors came, we'd peer surreptitiously to see who had come to visit our friends, and how warm or cool the relationship between them seemed to be. We all knew that when people are hospitalized, their close relationships must have been badly affected by the madness... When my family came to visit me, I always tried to put on a brave show in front of my buddies.

Suggestions

If I were a nurse on CPC2, there are some key things I would do differently.

First, I would make a point of coming out from behind the desk in the nurses' station at least once an hour, during which time I'd do a walk-around, check on my patients and simply be accessible to them.

Second, I would ensure excellent orientation for new patients. I was basically just steered to my bed and shown the washroom as we passed by. I was left to figure out all the rest for myself. What time are meals served? Where is the telephone and when can we use it? Where is the smoking room and what hours is it open? What occupational therapy sessions are offered and when? Are there any ward rules I should be aware of? All these and many more questions were churning in my misfiring mind. I wanted desperately to fit in, to be liked, and to be accepted by both the staff and patients. I was walking blind, with no cane to guide me. It was stressful not knowing what was expected, until much later when I had either solved the problem myself or simply imitated my fellow patients. I would therefore appoint veteran patients to be the official "greeters" and mentors for new admissions: each patient needs someone who can orient them to the ward, its functioning and rules, and introduce them to the other patients. This would help newcomers feel welcome and more relaxed from the start, promote a sense of community, and develop pride and leadership skills in the mentors. Failing this, a standard orientation for all new patients by a staff member would have been much appreciated.

Third, I would use mealtimes much more creatively to build a sense of community between patients – and staff – on the ward. Simple "community announcements" would have helped me to feel part of a group, rather than an isolated individual. For example: "Friends, today John is being discharged. I'm sure you all join me in wishing him the very best. [Applause for John.] And sometime this morning we will be welcoming a new patient, George. He will go into John's old bed. Please make him feel at home when you see him. Don't forget, today is our day to go swimming. Please wait by the elevator with your swimsuits and towels, ready to leave at 10 a.m. if you'd like to go swimming. Now, does anyone have any announcements or questions before we eat?" As one of my notes says:

> We live in community, but no community-building is done by the staff. We are members of a "lost-opportunity therapeutic community" – why does the staff NOT "build community" better?

Fourth, on the subject of food, although the meals were excellent, I was dismayed by the long gap between lunch at noon and dinner at around 5 p.m. No afternoon tea was served. I would have not only appreciated something warm to drink and some fruit, perhaps, but it would have been an uplifting break in the endless afternoon – something to look forward to between the interminable TV shows we all mindlessly watched. Even a coffee machine that we had to serve ourselves from, and pay for by the cup, would have been better than nothing.

Finally, I would put a suggestion box in a neutral place, not near the staff room where patients might feel intimidated about making anonymous suggestions. I'd empty the box regularly, and routinely encourage patients to submit suggestions. Every time a new admission arrived, I would re-announce the importance of the suggestion box. Depending on the suggestions received, I would read them out during community announcements time, and might even get a debate going to see if many patients agree with a specific suggestion or not. Empowering patients in this way would help them feel more engaged, responsible and in control, in a situation where they feel so infantilized and uprooted from their everyday lives.

~   ~   ~

Overall, my stay in CPC2 was very pleasant. I certainly expected far worse. In many ways, I felt like a passenger on a luxury cruise ship, with great food and plenty of leisure time. As far as I can recall, I was free to nap or shower at any time. The only things they asked us to do were to respect mealtimes and bedtime. It was, for the most part, quite relaxing (The Screamer excepted), secure, and sociable.

I didn't mind being there in the least.

Rob spent a lot of time begging the staff for permission to take me out, to go for a drive, a walk, or for a hot chocolate together. It was a victory when, right at the end of my stay in the hospital, we were allowed first to leave the grounds, and then go home for a six-hour pass, then an overnight pass, and eventually a weekend pass to see if the meds could control my moods back at home with all the stimulation there.

At home, I was advised to observe a "relatives only" policy for visiting and phone calls, as any over-stimulation might cause my mania to flare up again. I emailed all my family and friends to update them and received many loving replies.

When I was eventually discharged, I really felt safe. I've finally bridled this brute, I thought. Now, my job is just to return to normal, gently pick up the pieces and build a life that's balanced, controlled, stable.

Easier said than done.

Chapter 13: Relapse

During the three weeks between my two hospital admissions, my daily chart is largely blank. I just wrote:

> Asleep fourteen hours per night plus nap! No time
> to assess mood – mainly zonked out or neutral.

I was taking large doses of lithium, Epival, and Zyprexa. I saw my psychiatrist, Dr. R once a week, and she tweaked the dosages as necessary.

I was admitted for the second time on the morning of January 1, 2010. Four days before, I went hypomanic again. On the second day of that episode, I had a scheduled appointment with Dr. R, and she added Seroquel 50mg to my cocktail of meds in an effort to head things off. Unfortunately, that still wasn't enough to contain the mounting mania.

Normally, I am by no means a party animal, but around noon on December 31, I spontaneously and arbitrarily decided that we should host a New Year's party that very evening. Over the protestations of Rob and the kids, who were well aware that I was under strict orders *not* to get over-stimulated, I invited friends at short notice, and several who had no prior plans were delighted to accept. I was convinced that this was a first-rate idea and that the party would be a tremendous success. Mania had set in again, and I should have known better. But I was not yet familiar with my early warning signs so I waltzed blindly into mania's mean trap.

They say I was a control freak all night: ordering guests to come and play games whenever I decreed; snapping at some of the children in front of their trembling parents and other guests; constantly trying to amuse everyone and be the centre of attention throughout; and generally being both irritable and effusively charming by turns. How embarrassing.

Happy New Year!

As for me, I thoroughly enjoyed the party, but after all the excitement of cleaning the house, preparing food, and hosting, I was beyond exhausted. Yet I was too excitable to sleep. It wasn't long after the guests had left that I started misbehaving. The girls and Rob had consulted and all agreed that I would need to go back to the hospital to be assessed first thing in the morning. (We knew that Dr. R would – by sheer chance – be doing a shift in Emergency that day.) Strangely, I had no problem with that plan, and in fact started packing a bag, quite willing to go back and be re-admitted if necessary.

I have only spotty memories of the drama that transpired late that night, so the following description is based largely on what I have been told by Rob, Tami, Karrie and Karrie's friend who was visiting at the time. Thankfully, Matt was out at a sleepover that night, so he missed the ruckus.

Rob and the girls wanted me to stay upstairs and go to bed; it was so late it was early. But I insisted on going downstairs, wanting to email New Year's wishes to my family in South Africa. I also wanted to go outside as I'd done on several occasions before, wandering around town in the middle of the frigid night. Rob refused to let me near the door, knowing I'd try to bolt. So he blocked my way, which infuriated me. "I have a *right* to go out if I want to; you can't stop me! You're infringing on my human rights," I yelled. At one point, I rushed to the side door, planning to sneak out through the garage. When he stopped me, I cried, howled, accused him of imprisoning me. Then I tried to bargain sweetly: "Just for a short while; honest, I'll come straight back." I tried rationalizing, threatening, cajoling. Karrie heard all this drama from her bedroom upstairs, and realized it was going to be another long night. She made a makeshift bed on the floor by her door, where she could hear me better and react when necessary. She says that from about 3 to 5 a.m. I constantly tramped up and down the stairs, checking emails, trying to leave the house, and so on.

When Rob had stymied all my efforts to escape, I stomped upstairs and started phoning family members in South Africa to wish them happy New Year. Luckily, they are seven hours ahead of us, so I didn't wake anyone up. I was utterly charming on the phone, but when I saw Rob hovering nearby, I put my hand over the receiver and yelled: "F--k off – don't you dare try to unplug my phone!" To prevent him from unplugging it, I crouched down on my knees next to the wall and guarded the line like some cornered animal while continuing to dial numbers in South Africa. Sometimes, I even pretended to get through to someone and chatted away pleasantly, when in fact there was no one on the line! I alternated between speaking so plausibly and innocently to whomever I was calling and yelling at Rob to get lost. At last I stood up, and he firmly manoeuvred – pushed? – me down onto the bed, hissing: "You *have* to get some sleep now."

I was outraged at being manhandled, and kicked at him wildly, so he grabbed my foot to restrain me. I flailed viciously and kicked with my other foot. Again, he grabbed me to avoid being kicked. This unseemly tussle continued until I yelled: "Let me get up! Karrie, Tami, HELP; he's hurting me!"

Tami woke up first and staggered in. I was thrashing and screeching on the bed, with Rob clutching at my ankles, telling me to shut up and go to sleep, for God's sake. She confronted Rob: "Let her go!" and he retorted: "But she just won't keep quiet and go to sleep!" Then Karrie rushed in and pushed him away from me to the other side of the room.

Rob collapsed on a chair, defeated. He was utterly exasperated and exhausted. I accept now that any lack of self-control on his part was fully justifiable, but at the time I was extremely judgmental and mistrustful of him.

Yet another wedge between us.

When I was finally free, I jumped up off the bed and spitefully announced that I wanted to go back to the hospital where I'd be safe. I grabbed the phone to dial 911, but Rob quickly disconnected the phone. He had good reason: he had been told that when patients are brought in by their families or arrive voluntarily, the restrictions imposed in Emergency are less onerous than when they arrive by ambulance, and we had all agreed that Rob would drive me in the next morning.

I couldn't figure out why the phone wasn't working, so I went into the bathroom to use the phone in there. Again, Rob rushed in and disconnected it. I was too buzzy to plug the phone back in, so I just locked the door and started packing my toiletries for the hospital, humming happily to myself.

Happily? Sure: by then, the crazy mania spike had passed, and I felt quite peaceful.

When I emerged from the bathroom, I found poor Karrie and Tami slumped on the floor on the other side of the door, keeping close guard. "What are you doing out here, you maniacs?" I demanded judgmentally. The girls just looked at each other in disbelief – oh; so it's *we* who are maniacs? Ha!

Rob sidled towards me with a fast-acting Zyprexa pill that was supposed to calm me down, but I saw him coming and flatly refused to swallow it. I refused to have anything to do with him and waved him away imperiously, dismissively.

Seeing a small gap in their collective fortifications, I craftily made a sudden dash to the stairs. Everyone scrambled in hot pursuit. The girls held me back while Rob ran down to block the bottom of the stairs. They knew if I got downstairs, I'd be out of the door and gone into the night. They then tried to get me back up to bed, half-dragging, half-carrying me. I collapsed down on the stairs like a well-trained protester, deliberately trying to make myself heavier. I just wanted to get the hell out of the house, away from them all! Then I had a brilliant idea: one last chance at rescue. I yelled at the top of my voice for Karrie's friend, who was innocently trying to stay out of things in the basement guestroom, to come and help me. "Help! Help! They won't let go of me! *He-e-e-elp!*"

No luck. No help materialized.

This commotion on the stairs – yelling, pleading, tugging, shoving, collapsing, blaming – went on for too long. Finally, Karrie snapped and announced that she was going to call an ambulance. Rob was long past the end of his rope and didn't even try to dissuade her.

The police arrived first, then the ambulance. I was self-consciously well behaved with them and put on an elaborate show about being totally rational and reasonable. My manic spike had passed, and I convinced myself that I didn't really need to go back to hospital. I was sure I could persuade them that my family was mistaken about my mental state. I almost made myself sick, I was so sugary and fake with them.

Imagine my surprise when I found myself lying flat on my back in the ambulance with a kind young paramedic sitting opposite, making small talk. I guess I had been outnumbered. Or maybe my performance wasn't as convincing as I had thought. It didn't take long once we hit the highway for me to start fading out. Finally, my energy was spent. I slept until we got to the Emergency at the Douglas.

Ah; here we go again.

This time, I only stayed a few hours in the Emergency before being transferred back to CPC2. It felt like I had never been away. Some of the same patients from my first admission were still there. And at least this time I knew the routine; there was no stress trying to figure out how things worked. I settled back in contentedly.

It was such a relief to be on sabbatical from my annoying family. Damn them all!

My Seroquel dose was increased from 50 to 200mg, on top of lithium, Epival and Zyprexa. After about ten days, things settled enough for Dr. W to wean me out of the hospital, first with a six-hour pass, then a pass to sleep at home for one night, and finally a weekend, after which I never had to return except to clear out my cupboard and say my farewells.

No matter how close I had felt to some of the patients when I was one of them, now that I had been discharged, there was a palpable barrier between us: I was no longer one of "us" on the inside, I was one of "them" on the outside – one of those sane enough to be trusted out there.

I went home and started to pick up the pieces of my shattered identity in the aftermath of hospitalization.

Part 4:

Befriending bipolar

Chapter 14: Aftermath

My two psychiatric hospitalizations were peak moments; life-changing experiences; turning points in my illness. I expected that afterwards, all would be well; my wild moods would be controlled; I would get on with my life again.

No such luck.

It took over seven stormy months – until August 2010 – to achieve the cherished goal of stability. In the interim, there was the aftermath of hospitalization – with all its ups and downs – to survive.

Diary entries

During the period after my discharge, I kept a diary.

Monday, January 11, 2010
Today was my fourth day at home on an extended weekend pass. I feel totally calm – no irritable outbursts or exasperated moments, etc. I'M BACK! I am still sleeping in the basement to stay away from Rob, but spent all day upstairs, a lot of time at my desk, etc. Yay!!

But Rob flies to Iqaluit on Wednesday this week; will be gone for ten days. So the kids will have to cope on their own if I need hospitalization again. *Hrmph.*

Tuesday, January 12, 2010
Had a great day today: no signs of mania; functioned well and did some work with Rob. Woo-hoo!

That is literally the first work I have managed in many, many weeks – or should I say months? I'm slow, to be sure; and not everything thrills me (there's a huge backlog, etc.), but I will not let things get me down. I will be patient and respectful towards myself. I have just come out of hospital, after all... Need to rest and recuperate... no shame in that!

Was officially discharged today.

Will sleep downstairs again tonight: Rob and I are just too prickly with each other to be left alone yet.

We had a family meeting during dinner to clarify what to do in the event that I go manic in the middle of the night (sounds like a song or book title). Everyone seems clear about our game plan. But still: Dear God, please don't let me subject the kids to another bipolar episode while Rob is away.

Wednesday, January 13, 2010
Rob flew to Iqaluit, leaving very early.

Another great day. Tami and I went out for brunch and shopping at the health food store.

Decided to sleep in the basement again tonight: even with Rob gone, having me downstairs signals to the kids that I am not yet 100% confident in my recovery, and we all need to be cautious.

Friday, January 15, 2010
Went for follow-up appointment with Dr. R. She's happy to leave the meds as Dr. W prescribed in

CPC2. Nothing was said about sudden weight gain: the priority is obviously mental stability at this stage... Next appointment with her is in two weeks. She'll order blood tests then to check medication levels.

Saturday, January 16, 2010
Aha! First day I was in the office for a substantial period. Tidied desk, sorted through piles of paper. Hmm; is this a corner I'm finally turning? I hesitate to say it out loud; don't want to jinx it!

Spike of anger

My friend Navid reminded me of a nasty incident that happened one day shortly after my discharge when she and Leyla came with me to check out a wellness centre where Tami and I had gone for yoga and where a life coach worked. I wanted to sign up for life coaching sessions, but I wanted my friends' opinions of the coach before I did so. I was apparently so enthralled by the coach, I kept my friends waiting for ages. They came to find me after a while, but I said I was still busy talking. "Go for a walk or something," I snarled. They did. When they returned some time later, I was still totally engrossed with the coach. Navid asserted herself, and said: "Merryl dear, come. It's time to go now." Something snapped and I'm told that I screamed at her: "Navid! You can't rush me. I'm in the middle of something important here." She said the whole building shook with my shouting, and people working in the offices downstairs came to the stairwell to see what all the fuss was about.

My, my. A random spike of uncontrollable anger left over from my pre-hospital mania.

How embarrassing.

Ups and downs

Despite all the meds I was taking, I had another depression in late January and early February 2010, and a hypomanic episode in February – I had to sleep in the basement again for about a week. I sketched a brain with lightning bolts emanating from it, and wrote in the margin:

> Brain waves >> brain tsunami. Slept in the basement. Only had 3.5 hours of sleep.

Imagine how bad it might have been without all those meds tethering me down to reality. On February 9, I wrote:

> At last! I'm in the sweet spot! Slept in the basement to avoid fights with Rob. I was able to work for six or seven hours total. Feels like the cogs in my brain are finally intersecting.

To emphasize the point, I drew a primitive sketch of three cogs all working well together.

I sent an email update to friends and family, informing them about progress since I was discharged and attaching several photos from Christmas.

> Hi All,
>
> To all who have written recently and been left waiting much longer than usual for a reply: HI, THANKS for your patience and for prompting this reply.
>
> Rob has been working himself to the bone, trying to cover for me at work and in the family as well. I

don't know how he does it – my having bipolar when the two of us are the sole partners in a small business is really tough... I have been giving thought to other possibilities, but it's hard to change from our comfort zone and to think of selling this beautiful home Rob has designed and built for us.

How much easier it would be to cope with my illness if a) we had other partners in our company to share the load of covering for me or b) Rob had a job where we didn't work together. Then he would only have the stress of a sick wife to deal with; not a sick wife and a sick colleague too.

As for me, it's been huge drama for a few months now. I was in and out of the psychiatric hospital twice, taken in by ambulance both times, for a total of almost a month.

After all the drama, I am now on four major psychiatric meds (used to be on only one for the first year since diagnosis), so this is a huge change. We'll see if that settles things. Side effects are another story: I have put on 30 pounds in six weeks. And I need a full 14 hours of sleep every day, and even then, I get drowsy in the late afternoons. Not sure if I will be able to drive: that is being assessed as we speak. Not pleasant, but if this is what it takes to bring stability, I'll take it for sure.

Enough of me and bipolar. In other news...

Finally, on February 16, the hypomanic episode ended. I made a note that I slept upstairs all night, and got some good work done during the day. And same for the next day, and the two days after that. Then the chart is blank – always a bad sign, as that means I was so depressed I couldn't even bring myself to mark a little dot on my daily chart each evening.

And so the last week of February and the first two weeks of March 2010 were bleak times again. In the second week of April, another depression struck and lasted for two weeks. In early May, I was stable for about two weeks, followed by seven draining weeks of depression – again. In late June and early July, I was stable for about two weeks.

Follow-up appointment

During this brief respite in late June 2010, about six months after my second discharge, I go to see Dr. R for a routine follow-up appointment. In the waiting room of the Bipolar Unit, I see all kinds of people. Some walk briskly, upright, looking confidently straight ahead. They are either staff members or they are currently well. Lucky them. Lucky *us* – I am one of them, for now. Others might as well have a big sign around their necks: "I am in depression." Hair unwashed, uncombed, clothing wrinkled and dirt-stained, shoulders slouched, eyes glazed or averted, exhaustion and desperation oozing from them. I've been there, done that so many times, it gives me a chill to see that part of myself reflected in their unkempt appearances, their deflated postures, their pitiful anguish. I silently send out a little prayer for each one of them: "May it pass soon. May you find some relief." And for me: "Please, please; may my stability last."

In all these years, I've never seen a (hypo)manic patient in the outpatient waiting room. I guess they have either missed their appointments while they are out being wild and crazy, or they are in Emergency waiting for admission if things got too hairy. I've been there, done that, too.

I help myself to a water bottle from a large tray in the waiting room. I twist hard, and twist again before the cap finally snaps open. As I lift the thin plastic bottle to my lips, it clicks and cracks quietly. I drink hungrily and my upper lip is sucked down awkwardly into the neck of the bottle, creating a vacuum that releases itself noisily when I finally stop drinking. I immediately repeat this action, being parched from my old familiar lithium-thirst. What a relief to quench it!

I reflect that these water bottles have been provided, free, by the hospital for all the psychiatric patients like me who are on thirst-inducing medications. How sweet of them, I think. How considerate. Later, during my appointment, Dr. R informs me that all the water fountains are out of order, and because of the recent heat wave, they have decided to provide free water bottles to everyone. Just holding that small gift, that clear, fluid treasure in my hands makes me emotional. Someone cares. Someone understands what we need. I am respected here.

Despite everything, I am loved.

At this appointment, Dr. R says: "We're running after many rabbits: there's mood stability, weight loss, better sleep, ability to concentrate and work well, and so on. But the most important of all is mood stability. Do you understand that?"

I certainly do. And much as I would have loved to chase some – no, all – of those other rabbits, I am resigned.

She decides to wean me off Zyprexa and start Invega, a new anti-psychotic, instead. Lithium, Epival, and Seroquel are still on the menu, with occasional small dose changes over the following few months. Later, the Seroquel is stopped, and still later, the Invega as well. Now, I am only on lithium and Epival.

Achieving stability

Just a week or so after this appointment, I fell back into an-other six-week depression in July and August.

Then finally, after all these downs and ups, this is where I heave a belly-deep sigh of relief. From the last week of August 2010 to January 2016, I was stable.

S-T-A-B-L-E-!

For five-and-a-half years! Do you have any idea what that meant to me? If you are a fellow bipolar sufferer, I'm sure you do, especially if you have rapid cycling bipolar like I do. Each day of stability is a godsend I am deeply thankful for.

General side effects

I was put on so many different medications at different times that I found it hard to keep track of them all. To help me keep track, I made a spreadsheet with all the meds and their known side effects, and I then noted, using a scale of 1–10, which of those side effects I was experiencing, and to what extent.

I also asked Rob what changes he had noticed in me since I went on the meds. He mentioned slurred speech, hand tremors, swollen feet and ankles, weight gain and weakness. He said he found my gait to be uneven, using more of a left-to-right shuffle rather than a forward motion. My balance was also poor: I had to nervously clutch the handrail for fear of falling on the stairs. He also noticed my incomplete sen-tences; difficulty recalling; "lost words" (searching for words for common items, feelings, people, etc.); snoring; shortness of breath; and stiffness after mild exercise.

Tami, my main movie-watching partner, notes that I always used to weep unabashedly during sad movies, but now

I am emotionally detached or numb. It's true: this applies even to real life and family matters: I am one step removed from all the swirling human dramas playing out around me.

Scary.

Weight gain

When Cathy in CPC2 said she had gained 100 pounds in a year because of her meds, I found it very hard to believe. But even as we spoke, my own odyssey up the mountain of my weight chart had already begun. I weighed 136 pounds on October 25, 2009, having actually lost weight on lithium from 152 pounds. (Lithium can also cause weight gain but did not do so in my case.) Dr. R started me on Seroquel on October 20, 2009 because I was in depression. Weight gain began almost immediately. Then Epival and later Zyprexa were added, and I took off like a sprinter hungry (pun intended) for the finish line.

Somehow my meds had flipped on a previously unknown appetite centre in my brain. Eating became a major-time job. I still remember one morning after a generous breakfast, I put my dishes in the sink and, still feeling peckish, sidled to the pantry to see what might be worth eating. I started with almonds, by the fistful, eaten directly out of the large jar. Every now and then, I'd put the lid back on the jar, thinking, "That's enough now!" But the next thing I knew, the jar was gaping at me again and I was having "just one more" handful. And then another, and so on. Next, I found crackers. There was some cheese in the fridge. Say no more. Then, after all that savoury food, something sweet, perhaps? Peanut butter and honey on toast. Jam on more toast. Frozen waffles with maple syrup. Yum!

In this way, I gorged on, until I glanced at the kitchen clock, and saw that it was nearly time for lunch. Yay! At least now I could eat a meal with no guilt.

Now then, what's for lunch? I'm ravenous!

Somewhere in the back of my brain it struck me as abnormal that I had not left the kitchen for even a moment between breakfast and lunch and had been eating non-stop during those hours. But somewhere else, deep in my medicated brain, much stronger messages to "eat-eat-eat!" suppressed those responsible cautions.

I was chemically compelled to eat.

No surprises then: I gained between one to two pounds a week consistently for about nine months.

Good grief.

The peak of my obesity mountain was 192 pounds, 56 pounds above my starting weight.

The arches in my feet collapsed under the burden, so my heels buckled outwards in an unsightly manner, and my bunion got much worse, causing a hammertoe. I walked like a worn-out old woman, stiffly and self-consciously. My knees and thighs chafed against each other infuriatingly. My XXL then XXXL clothes stretched over my grossly enlarged bottom. My belly looked seven months pregnant. My chin was bloated like a toad and waggled when I talked. I could barely get up from sitting, my knees took so much strain. I bought elastic knee guards to help support the weight.

My ankles were swollen like overstuffed sausages. I was worried about my kidneys, and in March 2010, I went for a nephrology consult at the local hospital. The nephrologist laughed at me: he had seen so much worse in his time, he didn't care at all that my formerly slim ankles were now a source of utter embarrassment to me. The more weight I gained, the worse the swelling got. By July, I was paying for weekly lymphatic drainage massages, trying to reduce the unsightly and uncomfortable swelling in my legs. It took months for the swelling to subside, and even now, my fingers and ankles are not back to normal.

Getting in and out of the van was a laborious and awkward process that left me puffing from exertion.

I felt like a freak going to the community swimming pool, where I would thrash about, flailing desperately and gasping for air, until I finally accepted defeat, gave up even trying to swim – one of my favourite summer activities, normally – and just waddled around in the shallow end, trying to stay submerged up to my shoulders to hide my full size. I tried to exercise by huffing on our treadmill in the basement – which seemed to creak and buckle under my load – rather than going outdoors where normal-sized people would see me trying to work off some flab.

I hated myself in that state.

I have studied sociology, and always enjoyed observing people. Now that I had joined the ranks of the obese, I obsessively assessed other overweight people, trying to gauge whether they were better or worse off than me. When I saw someone who was lugging around even more dead weight than I was, I felt momentarily buoyed: "Ha! See, I'm not so bad after all!"

But then I'd look down at my massive belly and have to acknowledge the awful reality of my situation.

t of my fat-watching game was also: "I wonder if s/he is on meds, like me?" I'd try to read the signs to see if I could recognize fellow travellers in Bipolar Country. Either way, I felt new empathy for obese people. I had always been judgmental before; now I knew much better. We are people. We have feelings. We wish we didn't weigh so much. We'd give anything not to look like this.

Please don't judge us.

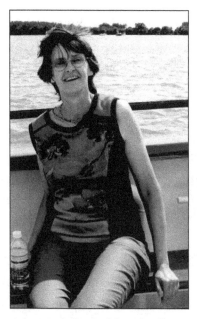

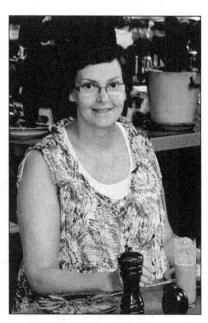

July 2008, before weight gain: slim face & upper arm; visible collar bone between necklace & t-shirt.

July 2010, after weight gain: full cheeks, neck, upper arm & belly; collar bones buried deep under fat. Funny that this photo was taken at the table!

Once I had peaked at 192 pounds, the disagreeable and extremely arduous descent down the other side of the weight chart began.

Pound by impossibly recalcitrant pound, I dieted and exercised my way back. It was excruciatingly slow. Sometimes I lost a pound a week – that was great. Other times, I got stuck at the same weight for several weeks at a stretch. That was really discouraging.

After over two years of focus and dedication, during which time Dr. R stopped the Zyprexa, Seroquel and Invega, I *finally* reached my starting weight again. What a relief! Staying at that weight now requires constant vigilance.

Sleep

All my life, I have loved to sleep. I liked getting seven or eight hours a night when I could, and more on weekends. I could happily doze for nine or ten hours as a treat. After being in hospital, I had no choice. The meds totally changed my sleep patterns; I needed much more than before. At the same time, they caused excessive thirst that then caused frequent urination, so my nights were maddeningly disturbed. Until my lithium dose was substantially decreased and I was drinking a bit less, I had to wake four or five times a night; now I'm down to once or twice, which of course is much better.

I chart my hours of sleep and naps on my daily chart, so I have detailed records of exactly how my sleep pattern has changed over the months. Or should I say, over the episodes and associated medication changes.

When I was depressed, I could barely sleep, and would lie awake for hours and hours, ruminating and anxiously re-thinking useless, dark thoughts. I would finally get between about four and six hours of sleep. Then I'd be so tired, and also want to hide from the world, so I'd have two, three, or even four naps, each lasting from fifteen minutes to an hour or so.

In (hypo)mania, on the other hand, I would be so buzzy that I could get by on zero sleep or just a couple of hours, and no naps at all.

During periods of stability, I used to sleep for about nine to eleven hours at night, and would, about half the time, have a nap lasting from half-an-hour to two hours during the afternoon as well. When my doses were reduced again, the afternoon naps all but stopped, and I now sleep eight to nine hours at night.

Libido

> "[Before bipolar:] The sex was/ Simply inspired./ Now there's no sex, she's depressed,/ And me I'm just tired./ Tired. tired. tired." *(sic)* ~Yorkey (2010:21)

Bipolar took a devastating toll on my libido and sex life. Was it the disorder itself? Side effects of the medications? The emotional impact of bipolar episodes on our marriage? The weight gain that sickened me and I assumed must make me appear repulsive to Rob? The hormonal impact of menopause that coincided with the emergence of bipolar in my case? Maybe all of the above. Regardless, bipolar sidelined sex.

In depression, sex was entirely out of the question. It would have been an affront to me, an outrage. I was inert, completely out of commission. The bed was weighed down with my woes; there was no way that sex – perky and frisky as she is – could have wriggled in there while I was in that utterly desolate state.

When I was hypomanic, my interest in sex was unusually heightened, but I felt eerily disconnected from myself and from Rob: not emotionally present, not intimate at all.

More recently, in stability, my libido is still largely lost in action. I am longing for a miracle. We live in hope.

About two years after hospitalization, I did a creative writing course. In one session, each participant made a collage from magazine pictures, and then wrote something about the collage. I chose pictures of couples doing fun and intimate things together: riding a tandem bike, eating in a restaurant, running on a beach, kissing in an ad for diamond rings, and so on. My accompanying text reads:

> I am a woman who's been blessed with genuine intimacy and closeness.
>
> Rob and I went everywhere together, arm-in-arm or holding hands, kissing every time the elevator doors closed, contriving never to spend a night apart so we could sleep together and wake together.
>
> I am a woman who longs to reclaim that intimacy.
>
> The shock of this illness and the side effects of my medications have run a sword between us, and we are both bleeding too profusely to take proper care of each other.
>
> I am a woman who longs.

Chapter 15: Back from the brink

"[Bipolar strikes] only because I was foolish enough to stumble into a place where I knew it lived. Bipolar disorder has territories." ~Presley (2010:133)

In Inuit folklore, *qallupilluit* are scary, witch-like creatures who live under the sea-ice and grab children who venture onto the ice without their parents. Inspired by the image of these evil beings, I think of bipolar as comprising two such creatures: "depression demons" who live under the earth and drag us deep down into a grave-like existence, and "mania monsters" who live up in the sky and pull us up-up-up so that when we eventually, inevitably fall back to earth, we crash really hard. Between these two feuding fiends, we are run ragged.

But here's the trick. Just as the *qallupilluit* wait for their prey by the cracks in the sea-ice, so the bipolar demons and monsters wait for us to stray off the straight path of recovery and remission. As long as we stay safely on the path, as intelligent, empowered and engaged bipolar patients, taking our meds, sleeping enough hours, eating well, exercising, meditating, not abusing drugs and alcohol, and using all the other self-care strategies outlined in Appendix 3, they will not be able to grab us. Well, no guarantees with this disorder. But surely they will grab us much less often than if we ignore all the guidance about self-care for stability.

As it happened, both "mania monsters" and "depression demons" tried to grab me within weeks of writing the above paragraphs about them back in 2010. They're out there, and we have to be super-vigilant to escape their clutches.

Fighting a hypomanic blip

The trigger for my hypomanic blip was a classical musical concert that Tami and I attended in November 2010. The music – by a trio that included a pianist – was flawless, sublime. But melodious music is not enough to spark an episode, surely. No, I believe it was the combination of the music and the powerful emotional connection I made between it and my beloved late Aunty Vee, my dad's sister, who used to teach piano lessons in my hometown of Johannesburg. I studied piano with her throughout my childhood, and all my life the piano has been intimately associated with her. These memories of my youth then stirred up the distant tugging of aching homesickness that every immigrant experiences on and off.

"Oh, I just *love* Mendelssohn!" I gushed to Tami on the way to the car after the standing ovation. "Did you see in the program that he was only thirty-eight when he died? I wonder why he died so young?" "Syphilis, I suppose," said Tami cynically. "All the great artists died of syphilis back then." That seemed too mundane for me. I thought maybe suicide. Who knows, I elaborated dramatically to myself, maybe he too had bipolar – well, manic depression as it was then called. As soon as we got home, I went online to research this point. Turns out it was a series of strokes that killed him. So he was not a kindred spirit after all; not "one of us."

How disappointing.

Rob called from the Arctic – where he was travelling for work – that night. He was away for several weeks and checked in with me at least once or twice a day. I found myself

nattering at high speed about the concert, and the tragic details of Mendelssohn's early death that I had researched, and
all kinds of random topics that simply occurred to me at the
time. I could feel myself speeding up, like a wind-up toy released onto the floor. I caught myself: "Oh-oh, I need to slow
down a bit," and told Rob that I should end the conversation
– monologue? – so I could take a quiet bath and get to bed at
a reasonable hour. I didn't confess: "I feel a bit fizzy." He was
so far away and I didn't want to worry him. But I did indeed
feel fizzy, and it frightened me rigid.

I ran a bath, lit a candle, and relaxed there, breathing
deeply and mindfully for a while. It felt like my pulse was racing and my breathing was speeded up, but when I checked
these vital signs, both were in fact on the slow side. Odd! But
there was a bubbly feeling in my stomach: a mixture of thrill,
anticipation and joy. I knew this elated feeling only too well
from previous hypomanic episodes. Breathe deeply. Just relax
and breathe…

I added more hot water and relaxed back against the
bath pillow. Ah; this is the life. But then, suddenly, I stopped
and stared, blinking in disbelief and terror. Curling wisps of
steam were rising from the water and swirling upwards. No
sooner had one wisp evaporated than another emerged.
Sound familiar? Remember the visual hallucinations on my
birthday back in 2009 when I saw steam rising from all the
trees?

Oh no; am I hallucinating again?

Whew! I realized what was happening: the steam was
in fact real – rising from the hot water in the bath. Just as
you'd expect. I was not hallucinating or imagining anything.
It was only that the candlelight from the edge of the bath

caused the steam to be clearly visible compared to every other night when I only turn on a dim light in the bathroom and the steam rises unseen.

What a relief!

After my bath, I took a prescribed sleeping pill to ensure a solid night's sleep – essential for hypomania prevention. Thankfully, I slept well.

The next morning, I informed the kids what was going on ("I'm in hypomania-prevention mode") and did a relaxing session of meditation before breakfast. I moved and talked very self-consciously, deliberately slowing myself down, reining myself in. I was walking on eggshells, and if one broke, it wouldn't just be egg on my face: I might end up back in hospital.

After lunch, I went for a stroll in the nearby woods with Karrie, Tami and some friends. It was so relaxing to be outdoors enjoying the fall leaves. Then it was time for exercise. I decided to do some gentle yoga instead of going on the treadmill as usual. Yoga is more calming, more suited to my program of "bring me down before I fly off into mania again."

At dinnertime, we had CBC radio on and Randy Bachman's *Vinyl Tap* show was featuring drummers. I was enjoying it immensely and found myself wanting to dance along. Oh no. Way too stimulating for me, so we switched that off, and I did another meditation session instead. We then watched a romantic comedy (no action or drama to over-stimulate me), and I went to bed early again.

Were these precautionary steps enough to nip this potential episode of hypomania in the bud? Thankfully yes.

Within two days, I was 100% back to normal. Mission accomplished. Emergency – quite literally – averted.

This is how I think about hypomania prevention: I have fire smouldering in my brain. It's under control at the moment, thank goodness, but it could rage up again at any time if I'm not vigilant about my self-care program. This time, there were two little twigs in my brain, ignited by my over-emotional reaction to the classical music concert. Luckily, I heard the snapping and cracking of the fire starting and smelled the smoke immediately. At once, I made a wide perimeter around the blaze: I meditated, had a candlelit bath, took a sleeping pill, went to bed early, informed my family, did yoga, and so on. No new twigs were added to the fire: no over-stimulation, no stress, no late nights, no drugs or alcohol, no missed doses of meds, no self-blame. Within two days, the little fire had completely burned itself out, leaving hardly any ashes to sweep up.

That first aid kit served me well for hypomania prevention. I wondered if I'd be able to prevent a relapse into depression as effectively.

Fighting a depressive blip

As it turned out, I didn't have to wait long to prevent a depression emergency. About a month later, one Saturday afternoon in mid-December 2010, I got some deeply upsetting news about a dear family member. Within minutes of hearing the news, I thought: "Oh dear, this is precisely what could trigger a depression. I'd better be vigilant." I monitored my mood more closely than usual, and for the rest of that day and the whole of Sunday, I felt fine. "Thank goodness; false alarm," I thought. But on Monday morning, sitting in the rocking chair where I do my meditation, I felt a well-known ache in my stomach. I felt glued to the seat by that awful leaden feeling that makes any movement too arduous to contemplate, let alone perform. I also started yawning incessantly: I was utterly overcome by a deep, gnawing exhaustion. Sleep was the only thing on earth that interested me.

All this felt very familiar, of course, and I would do anything not to go down "depression road" again.

Shamelessly, I lectured myself: "You have a choice to make here, woman. Either curl up in bed and hope that things will improve on their own or take an active role and try to change the way you feel right now, before it gets any worse." Buoyed by my recent success in beating the hypomania blip, I decided on the latter approach.

I forced myself up from the chair and tottered into the kitchen to clean up a bit. Just the small movements to wipe down counters and put dishes away shifted my headspace a bit. I felt a distinct lightening of mood. Thank goodness! Next, I took a radical (for me, at that time of the day) step: go downstairs and climb onto that dreaded treadmill ("Dreadie Treadie" as I call it) and get my heart rate up for a while. I couldn't trot as fast as I normally do, and I couldn't keep going for as long as I like to, but I did it. Fifteen minutes of brisk walking and I felt like a new woman. Not only the exercise but the sense of accomplishment cheered me.

In my bipolar therapy group, we had been told: "You can change your posture and physiology to change your thoughts and mood." For example, stand up from lying on the bed; walk to the window to look outside. Straighten your shoulders. Lift your chin, look up at the sky, and smile! It's well worth a try.

For me, that's all it took that time: a conscious decision to fight, movement in the kitchen, and some moderate physical exercise. Had I needed more intervention, I would have listened to loud, cheerful music; watched a comedy show or amusing YouTube clips; read my list of wonderful and funny things that have happened in my life; sung; danced; spent time with friends who make me smile and laugh; and so on.

Another trick I learned in my therapy group is to set small goals to get the frontal lobes of the brain working. They said this brain activity helps to challenge the depression. So: "First, I am going to take a shower. Then I'll get dressed. Next, I will eat something healthy. After that, I will write in my journal, then phone a friend to chat…"

Baby steps.

Just keep putting one foot in front of the other.

Preventing both hypomania and depression

Some interventions are common to both hypomania and depression prevention: take your medications faithfully, keep a detailed daily self-care chart and journal (see Appendix 2), learn to recognize your early warning signs, get good sleep (but not too much sleep when depressed – ten hours maximum), eat well, meditate, avoid alcohol and drugs, use stress reduction and relaxation techniques, and keep a hopeful and positive attitude. As mentioned, I elaborate on all these strategies in Appendix 3.

I hope that some of these suggestions will help you bring yourself back from the brink next time you feel the first early signs of an impending (hypo)manic or depressive blip. Or, better still, motivate you to think of strategies that might work even better for you.

Imagine if we could prevent full-blown bipolar episodes by being vigilant and dedicated to our self-care programs.

Relapse and recovery

If you were reading closely in Chapter 14 when I addressed the issue of *Achieving stability*, you might recall this sentence: "From the last week of August 2010 to January 2016, I was stable." But it's now over two years later.

What happened in January 2016, you ask?

It was all my fault. Preventable.

Rewind to summer 2015. After five full years of stability, both Rob and I agreed that it would be worth trying to wean me off my meds. We were concerned about possible side effects from long-term use. I knew that Dr. R would never have agreed to this plan, but she was on leave at the time, and the psychiatrist replacing her gave his blessing for a weaning trial, cautioning me that a relapse was entirely possible.

Of course, I knew that I was taking a risk, but it seemed worth a try.

It took six full months to cautiously wean off both Epival and lithium under this psychiatrist's supervision, and I finally had three glorious weeks without any meds whatsoever.

I felt much more productive, clear-headed, and "just myself."

So happy!

I wrote in my journal:

19 November 2015

Been off lithium for ages now, and off Epival since 8 November. So far, so good! I feel great!

Clearer mentally; more alert. Sleeping better than usual. Doing meditation and exercise faithfully. You go, girl!

Then with no warning, one morning I felt "off." Depression descended. I could *not* believe it.

I tried every trick I knew to fight back. After three days I had to admit defeat and call the bipolar clinic for an urgent appointment. I need meds!

Here we go again…

I was immobilized for a miserable month before the meds kicked in, or the depression just faded.

Now, nearly ten years after my initial diagnosis in 2008, I am once again stabilized on lithium and Epival. In Appendix 3, I reflect in detail on the self-care techniques I use to maintain this stability in conjunction with my meds.

After that relapse in January 2016, I had to re-start counting my weeks and months of episode-free living. Like an alcoholic who relapses after many years of sobriety and has to start from zero again.

Today, I'm up to twenty-six months.

And counting.

Chapter 16: Gains and losses

If you had asked me years ago, before I got sick with bipolar, how I would feel if I were ever diagnosed with a mental illness, my response would have been immediate and categorical. Unthinkable! Disastrous! End of the world!

Of course, there have been some major challenges – for me personally, and equally so for Rob and the children. But to my continuing surprise, not only has my world kept going around, there have even been some distinct benefits.

Let's ask: looking back, what have I gained and lost since becoming ill?

Gains

Balance at work

Bipolar has been something of a blessing in disguise. It's forced me to become more balanced and reasonable about the amount of work I do. Even more importantly, I am now realistic about what I expect of myself as a recovering workaholic. I am truly satisfied with a seven- or eight-hour workday most days; I don't feel guilty about "slacking off" for not working twelve, fourteen or even sixteen hours a day. I know that if I do more work, some crucially important aspect of my recovery plan will suffer: either I won't have time to exercise, or meditate, or relax, or get enough sleep.

I'm simply not prepared to put my mental health at risk for an extra couple of hours in my office.

Healthy lifestyle

Commitment to self-care and all the elements of a healthy lifestyle have immeasurably improved my life since I got bipolar. Now that I meditate every day, do regular exercise, sleep enough hours, and so on, I can't imagine ever having lived without practising these health-protecting measures.

Self-discipline

I now lead a rather regimented life. It takes self-discipline to get to bed on time, wake up on time, eat on time, exercise regularly, meditate daily, swallow my medications at the correct time every single day, and so on. For someone who was previously largely undisciplined – except where work was concerned – I count this as a major bonus.

A new perspective on mental illness

I'll reflect on this point a bit further in the final chapter, so I'll just say that when I "crossed the floor" from being mentally healthy to mentally ill, my entire perspective on mental illness changed radically. I am now – and always will be – "one of *them*." And – after eventually accepting my new identity – proud to be so.

Ability to "play the bipolar card"

> "I have used [bipolar] as an excuse for countless offensive behaviors." ~Presley (2010:133)

I can "play the bipolar card" at any time. For example, if I don't want to go somewhere, I can tell my family it will stress or overstimulate me too much; or if I don't want to work on something, I can tell Rob I need to rest. However, the joke is mainly on me, as there is more than an element of truth in these excuses: I simply can't function at the same pace as I used to, either because of the meds, or the disorder, or both.

Losses

While I am perfectly serious about the fact that I feel I have gained things since bipolar struck, it's equally true that I have also lost a lot.

My assurance of mental stability

Before bipolar, I never gave a second thought to my mental wellness. I took it totally for granted. Now, I will never – for the rest of my life – be able to shake the fear that I might relapse at any time. As I wrote in my journal in 2011:

> I seek, beyond all else, mental stability. Normalcy. Sanity. Back to the way I was before I made myself so dismally ill. I am worn out with the dread that I will relapse either into depression (God help me) or mania (God help everyone else). I hate nervously assessing my mood each day: "How am I feeling today? Am I too high, too low, or – please, please – just right?" Like some desperate version of Goldilocks always seeking the sweet spot...

My stigma-free identity

Having the label "bipolar" sets me apart from all my family and friends; mental illness is still – I don't care what you say – severely stigmatized in our society. I'm "mad" now.

It's not only society that stigmatizes mental illness, it's us – the sufferers – as well. I felt somehow guilty and ashamed when I was first diagnosed, as if I'd let myself – and my family

– down in some way. As I left Dr. Y's office in utter disbelief that fateful day, weighed down by the shocking new burden of my bipolar diagnosis, I looked away, hoping that passersby would not see what a leper I was. What a blow to my sense of identity. Wasn't I somehow "better" than this; "above" this?

Clearly not. I need to keep reminding myself:

> "I may have bipolar disorder, but I don't let it define me. Don't let it define you." ~Pilkington (2010:172)

My self-esteem

> "… I didn't realize that my old self was already gone forever. I didn't know yet that my career, my relationships and my health would be forever changed."
> ~McPheron (2010:50)

I used to feel competent, reliable and respected. A trustworthy adult citizen. All that changed with my diagnosis. The ground beneath me heaved and I lost my balance. I could no longer rely on my own brain. I couldn't implicitly trust my own judgments. I can't get through a single day without psychotropic medications. It sucks.

My productivity

Before I was diagnosed, my academic and professional productivity were critical to me. I was a successful public health consultant working on many interesting and intellectually challenging projects. I was a high-functioning, super-efficient, competent, socially outgoing person quite at ease in situations that required leadership. I put all my creative energy into my work – volunteer or paid – and loved every minute of it. Whatever project I undertook, I did with meticulous attention to detail.

Overnight, I was floored, my mental capacity rendered useless. In depression, I was in such a thick, oppressive fog I couldn't even check emails; in (hypo)mania, I was whizzing around in a glorious whirl – and sometimes in a far-from-glorious state of irritability – with work being the very last thing on my hyperactive mind. Now I had to accept that my brain – the mother of all organs – had become suddenly unreliable, unsound, unpredictable.

It was a jarring jolt. I had to learn that my brain needed care and attention to recover and permit me any level of normal functioning again.

Bottom line: we cannot ever take our brains for granted.

I am now considerably less productive than before the diagnosis. I still pay close attention to quality, but not to the obsessive degree I used to, and I am satisfied with a more modest output, consistent with the more reasonable number of hours I now work. I think of it as work on a human scale, rather than the super-human scale I used to demand of myself. I'd love to push myself, but I know the potential cost, so I don't. Well, most of the time, anyhow.

How responsible, how safe; but how dull, how boring.

My financial security

My income used to reflect the excessive professional efforts I made. I felt totally financially secure, confident that I would be able to continue working at that pace in the future.

Bipolar totally knocked that sense of security.

Since regaining my stability, I have been able to work again – "like a normal person". While this is obviously good news, it was a long time before I made up for the many lost months when I generated no income at all.

My unusually close relationship with Rob

Rob and I had always been incredibly close – best friends, equal partners and companions not only in life, but at work as well. He had always treated me with the utmost respect. Bipolar was a wedge hammered between us on all fronts, rendering me unpredictable, unreliable, and needing care, and transforming him from a calm, competent and trustworthy partner into someone I experienced as short-tempered, judgmental, and patronizing when I was (hypo)manic.

I wrote this journal entry in 2011:

> Rob, I have waited a long time to tell you how very thankful I am for your tender care and ministrations while I was so sick. I pray that you knew it all along, even when I was so self-absorbed and ungracious. You were a real advocate and companion every step on the way. I could not have managed without you, love. But at the same time, I have to tell you that I occasionally felt patronized by you. You talked down to me; bossed me; tried to prescribe courses of action that I insisted on resisting. I hated those times. At some level, I hated *you* at those times. Ouch.

What I hated was that I no longer felt equal: I was much more dependent on Rob, and that rocked my identity. Our emotional and physical intimacy was eroded: we treated each other in a much more business-like, fraternal way.

There was also a basic loss of trust: Rob could no longer rely on me the way he used to, either as a wife and companion, or as a co-worker; and I could no longer rely on him to remain consistently steady under extreme pressure. Having seen him lose his cool with me several times during manic episodes, I had to re-learn to fully trust him again. That loss of trust permeated every aspect of our relationship, spreading hairline cracks through the concrete, weakening the entire structure. And once some small distance came between us, it was easier to allow more remoteness to creep in, dividing our once inseparable couple-unit into two discrete individuals, both longing for close connection, strength and unity once more.

No wonder that even after all these years of complete stability, we are still clawing our way back to normalcy in our relationship.

Aspects of my role as a mother

As the (step)mother of five children, I was used to having their loving respect. Since becoming ill, I feel that I lost a lot of that closeness and respect, and that the kids – except for Kai, who lives too far away to be too much affected by this – actually tended to parent me in subtle and not-so-subtle ways.

They assumed the adult role and treated me more like an unreliable teenager than a competent parent. Menu planning for the week? They consulted together and informed me of their decisions. Social plans? Same thing. I was more the passenger, less the driver of the metaphorical bus. Matt observed that after I became ill, I became more of a "viewer" and less of a "do-er."

Tami has been my faithful companion on my bipolar journey: she was my exercise buddy; she took me clothes shopping in the plus-size stores when I gained weight; she supported me in whatever I proposed to do to stay healthy. I was extremely grateful for her support, but at the same time, some of her caring actions made me feel mothered by her, and this tended to reinforce my loss of credibility as a parent.

I used to complain a lot about being patronized by the kids when I was manic. I would yell at Rob: "They're patronizing me again. Keep them away from me – I can't stand the way they treat me! I won't put up with it!" (But I would also say that Rob was patronizing me, sometimes. I'd spit: "Stop patronizing me! I'm not a child!" That was one of my favourite things to say.)

Of course, the kids felt they were merely stepping in to fill the vacuum bipolar had created. It was never their intention to patronize me.

Mika observed that around the onset of my disorder, the youngest kids were all moving into early adulthood and she noticed that they were becoming more assertive and taking on more responsibility – not just with me but in all aspects of their lives. So perhaps what I interpreted as patronizing behaviour was in fact just them being more grown-up and self-assured.

Aspects of my friendships

My relationships with friends also shifted when I got sick. With them, it was subtler than with family members with whom I lived, but I still perceived a change. It was as if I were no longer an equal partner in the relationship, but rather a "younger," less responsible, less reliable version of myself.

Friends felt free to lecture me, much as they would one of their adult children, about what I should do to get out of depression, for example. I remember thinking: "If only you knew how patronizing this feels, you wouldn't preach at me like this."

While a few things like that irritated me, luckily our friendships were strong enough to withstand the tensions, and in general I felt their love and support through the whole drama.

My faith

My faith – the Baha'i Faith – had been a deeply significant part of my identity for about thirteen years before bipolar arrived. Then, within a matter of days, it was put out to pasture and left to fend for itself. Weeds entangled it, and it was soon entirely smothered. Before long, I wasn't able to say prayers for myself, let alone for anyone else.

I had been intensely active in the Faith before bipolar. I taught a children's class in our home every Friday evening. That now stopped. I participated in a series of study circles. No more. We hosted weekly junior youth meetings on Sunday afternoons. Enough. And I attended various devotional gatherings. *Adieu.*

Travelling through Bipolar Country took all my energy. My faith and spirituality got sidelined. Just when I needed them most.

Even now, many years of stability later, I still haven't regained my former fervour; I have less spiritual fire than before. I pray that as my recovery deepens, I will rediscover my spiritual strength and stop being a mere shadow of my former self.

My ability to react normally to events

Nobody ever warned me that people with bipolar often become hypersensitive to loud sounds and other jarring events. Or that we may over-react to everyday happenings and find it much harder than most to return to "normal" after any kind of a crisis.

I wish they had.

I often end up scaring *myself* with my over-the-top, completely out-of-proportion reactions.

A few examples. I'm looking out of the kitchen window when Rob or one of the kids walks into the room without my hearing them. They then cough, or put down a mug, or whatever, and I leap into the air, terrified, and scream blue murder: *Aargh!* Or if I'm alone in the house and the phone or doorbell rings, I startle and shout out in shock. And even as I do this, some deep part of my brain is critically assessing my irrational panic and *tut-tutting* at me: What's *wrong* with you, woman?

And yet, paradoxically, while I over-react in some situations – especially those that involve fear or surprise of some kind, I under-react to others – especially those that involve other emotions. I have lost much of my normal emotional connectedness. I've mentioned the emotional numbing I felt when my mom died. I also used to be known for my weepy reactions to sad movies, or tragic news reports. No more. My tears have dried up.

Who or what has turned down my emotional thermostat?

I used to live life in full technicolour; now it's sepia.

My normal weight

Loss of my normal weight hit me harder than I ever would have thought possible, and had negative ramifications for my physical health, identity, self-esteem, and my relationship with Rob. When I gained so much weight so suddenly, I asked the children if they were embarrassed by or ashamed of my weight. They assured me no; they realized the weight gain was due to the meds, and they saw how hard I was trying to lose the weight.

Me? I was both acutely embarrassed and profoundly ashamed.

Freedom to be spontaneous and adventurous

Another major loss is that I can no longer be young-and-fun, making spontaneous plans and participating in carefree adventures. I now live an almost monastic life, retiring to bed at more-or-less the same time every night, rising at more-or-less the same time every morning, and so on. Shall we take a weekend trip to the mountains? Well, it sounds wonderful, but will I be in bed by 11 p.m.? Shall I travel with Rob to the Arctic to work on our research project? Well, I'd love to, but they are two time zones behind us, and in the winter, they get virtually no daylight there. It could be risky for my stability.

Given my commitment to stability, I willingly err on the side of caution. Yes, I miss out on a lot, but not nearly as much as I'd miss out on if I have an episode again. My agendas for 2008, 2009 and 2010 are full of events that I had hoped to attend but cancelled due to either depression or mania: conferences, meetings, museum exhibitions, concerts, outings, social engagements, and so on. I even had to drag my depressed self to both Tami and Matt's high school graduation ceremonies. I felt like a washed-out remnant of myself observing the proceedings, all maternal pride and emotion buried deep by the mental fog.

~   ~   ~

When I look back at the kind of life I was leading – and role-modelling for our children – before I got bipolar, I am frankly ashamed. I'm a nurse, and I should have known better. My life was so far from balanced it's a wonder I didn't get sick sooner.

Now, I take pride in constantly seeking balance, and I know this benefits me not only mentally, but physically as well. And, as a bonus, I hope that our adult children will learn from my experience and eventually make similar commitments to their own health as well.

So in a way, getting bipolar was a backhanded godsend.

As I wrote in my Creative Writing class in 2011:

Getting bipolar disorder was obviously a shock and a real ordeal at the time. But it has also been a gift of sorts. I have learned patience, humility, self-control, obedience (compliance), and gratitude for previously taken-for-granted mental stability.

~   ~   ~

Consider: having bipolar is like being in an arranged marriage. You didn't choose this particular life partner, but now you're stuck with it. So, you can dwell on all the negatives and losses and be miserable your entire life, or you can focus instead on the positives and gains and feel blessed.

It's your choice.

Chapter 17: Emotional reactions

When I look back on my emotional reactions to being diagnosed with bipolar, and eventually learning to live with it, I see it's been a long and challenging journey.

I knew about the five stages of grieving proposed by Elisabeth Kübler-Ross (denial, anger, bargaining, depression, acceptance), but my own odyssey of grieving the loss of my mental health was considerably more convoluted than that. There was some overlap, for sure, between my stages of grieving and those of Kübler-Ross, but perhaps because of the stigma of mental illness, or perhaps because of my own weird psychological complexities, I needed to work through many more than five stages.

See which of these fourteen stages ring true for you.

Stage 1: Shock and disbelief

> "Mental illness is a thief, one that sneaks in and steals the beautiful painting of the life you've imagined for yourself…" ~McPheron (2010:49)

I've described my initial emotional reactions to bipolar in earlier chapters. It was my personal tsunami: I felt cruelly bowled over by a tidal wave. I lost my bearings and was swept way out to sea. I couldn't fathom any way of struggling back to shore safely.

I felt utter shock and disbelief.

Stage 2: Denial and rejection of the diagnosis

In classic Kübler-Ross style, I went into denial about having bipolar, and initially rejected the diagnosis.

Stage 3: Acceptance of the diagnosis and relief

> [When I was given the diagnosis:] "... I felt a faint glimmer of hope as I realized that at last we might have found what was really wrong with me." ~McPheron (2010:51)

When I finally accepted the diagnosis and the fact that I needed psychiatric treatment, there was a feeling of deep relief. Aah; so there's a good reason for all my strange feelings and behaviours. There's a rational explanation. I'm not to blame. I'm sick. And with treatment, I can surely improve.

Stage 4: Shame

Mental illness is still severely stigmatized. At the time of my diagnosis, I was still an offender in this regard. As a health professional, the offence of stigmatizing mental illness makes me doubly guilty. I really should have known better.

When I finally accepted my diagnosis, I had to deal with the shame of suddenly being identified as "one of them" – a member of the harshly judged and marginalized group of mental patients.

Stage 5: Pain and guilt

The biggest pain I suffered was caused by my loss of identity – discussed in the previous chapter.

> "[P]erhaps the best advice I can share is to remind yourself that bipolar disorder is a disorder – just that

– and that you should not let it define you. After all, have you ever heard anyone say, 'I am high blood pressure' or 'I am diabetes'?" ~McKinstry (2010:116)

My guilt was over things I hadn't done for my family when I was ill, and over what I was putting them through with my bipolar episodes. There was also the guilt of having "brought" a mental illness into the family, and with it, the fear that my disorder might one day affect my children, or theirs.

Stage 6: Self-consciousness

"When I felt good, I asked myself if I felt too good. When I felt sad, I asked myself if I was becoming depressed. Because I was constantly asking myself what and how I felt, I never really felt anything except confusion and worry." ~Whetsell (2010:58)

I constantly tried to monitor my behaviour: am I behaving appropriately for this situation? Am I laughing too loudly? Can I mask my depression a bit?

A poignant example of this second-guessing myself was evident after a party in August 2008, just days after my initial diagnosis. I had told my friends about my diagnosis, and wanted feedback from them about how I had behaved at the event. I emailed:

Since all of you know about my recent diagnosis, I thought I could ask you how I seemed to you tonight, so I can give some feedback to my psychiatrist when I see him again on Tuesday. Did you find me any different from my 'normal' self? Was I unusually hyper or socially inappropriate at all? Did I offend anyone – well, any more than I normally would have, anyway?!

All of them responded, and reassured me that I had, in fact, behaved "appropriately." But as one insightfully replied: "This must be so tough on you – to be analyzing your every move and wondering if it is within normal range or not."

Damn right it was!

Stage 7: Anger and bargaining

This stage was typical Kübler-Ross: Why me? Why now? If I seek every kind of help available, will I be cured?

Stage 8: In limbo

During both depression and (hypo)mania, I felt like I was in a mental, emotional, social and spiritual limbo, floating root-less. I wasn't me. It was as if I had been taken over by some obnoxious stranger who colonized and inhabited my body and my precious brain. It was outrageous, but it was my real-ity. And for as long as that went on, I was stuck in limbo.

Stage 9: Loneliness and rumination

In depression, I isolated myself as much as possible. I felt so bad I couldn't face socializing. And besides, I couldn't bear to inflict myself on my friends. As if I didn't want to "infect" them with my desperate mood. Then I'd spend hours mulling over my former life, ruminating about all that might have been if only the disorder hadn't struck.

Stage 10: Faked acceptance of the illness

Before the true acceptance that only came later, I experienced a stage of faked acceptance. I went through all the motions of being a "good patient," but deep inside I was still kicking and screaming at the universe for landing me in this mess. I took my disorder personally. I only tried to make people think I had accepted it so as not to appear immature or petty. After all, who did I think I was: so special that I should be exempted from the curveballs that life throws at all of us, at one time or another?

So, inwardly raging, I put on a brave, fake face.

Exhausting!

Stage 11: Resignation and adaptation

Gradually, I resigned myself to my new reality and started to genuinely adapt myself to it, instead of pining for my pre-bipolar reality. I had to build a new life that was compatible with the limitations imposed by the disorder. For example, I needed to take my meds, work fewer hours, exercise, and so on.

Stage 12: True acceptance and hope

> "Amanda's mental illness is not who she is, but only one facet of a multi-faceted, multi-talented human being with much to contribute to this world." ~Weil (2010:91)

Reality sinks in. I see bipolar as just one part of the whole me, not some monstrous imposter. I start to plan for the future, with bipolar as a full partner in that future.

Unless, of course, they find a cure for it one day!

Stage 13: Resilience

> "I am as resilient as an elastic band stretched to the
> limits of sanity, continually springing back to reality."
> ~Richards (2010:136)

In the past several years, I have bounced back and feel like my old self, only better in many ways. I'm not trying to sugarcoat the problems, such as medication side effects, but as I have explained there are many gifts this disorder has brought me.

Stage 14: Pride

By the time I decided to write about my experiences, I felt a certain pride: I had looked down the barrel of the bipolar gun and survived. I have stories and ideas to share. Maybe by speaking out, I can have some small effect on reducing the stigma attached to bipolar and other mental illnesses?

Recall my post-it from when I was first manic back in 2009. It read, in typically truncated style: "Civil rights. Women's rights. Gay rights. Mental health rights. Mad rights?"

I'm serious. We've had all those other great movements. Isn't it time for a mad rights movement? We should not have to hide in the closet just because we have a mental illness. We can look people square in the eye. We deserve respect and understanding.

May we all get past the understandable but unhelpful early stages of shock, denial, and shame when stigma clouds our judgment, and reach the stages of true acceptance, resilience, and pride – sooner rather than later.

~   ~   ~

Stages of grieving for loved ones and carers

It strikes me now that many of these same stages of grieving might apply to the family members, friends and carers of bipolar sufferers.

When the diagnosis is first given, they may experience shock and disbelief; denial and initial rejection of the diagnosis; acceptance of the diagnosis and relief that there is a logical explanation for the person's uncharacteristic behaviour; shame because of the stigma of mental illness; guilt in case the illness was somehow caused or worsened by them; self-consciousness about being associated with a mentally ill family member; anger and bargaining; loneliness and rumination about how life used to be before the strain of coping with a mental illness in their loved one; and even faked acceptance. Then, during the process of their gradually coming to terms with their new reality, they may feel resignation and adaptation; true acceptance and hope; resilience; and finally pride to be openly supporting and accepting someone with a mental illness.

~   ~   ~

One of my friends reflected on her reaction when I was first diagnosed. She felt she was not a good friend to me as I went through all my early bipolar dramas. She was frankly scared to visit me in hospital; she didn't want to face my reality head-on like that. She apologized for her "cowardice." She couldn't really explain why it happened – just the huge stigma and wanting to avoid the harshness of a mental illness, she supposed. "Forgive me for being such a fair-weather friend," she said.

Of course I forgave her! If *she* had become mentally ill, and I was still well, I would probably have reacted exactly the same way. It's only now that I have joined the ranks of the mentally ill myself that I feel comfortable opening up to others with – and without – a mental illness.

It shouldn't be that way.

Experts say that one in five people experiences a mental illness every year. That's a huge number. Engaging openly and positively with mentally ill people should be a normal part of life, a fundamental social skill. Something we don't even think twice about.

We have such a long way to go, so much educating to do.

It's an exciting challenge for us all.

Chapter 18: Final thoughts

Old life; new life

In the early days, it was a constant effort to regain and reclaim my mental health. It started as a daily struggle to follow my self-care routine. Gradually, that struggle became more manageable. Now, it's just the way I live. It's a small price to pay to keep myself stable. If I don't manage my own bipolar, who will?

I often think about my old life. But with much less regret now than before. Who's to say that my old life was any better than my new life? Was that really the best self I could be? Working 24/7, running myself ragged, neglecting so many other aspects of life in the process.

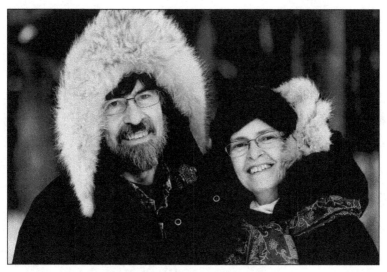

Almost back to normal; building a new life.
Taking a walk in the woods with Rob, February 2014.

I am more fulfilled and having more fun now, with this diagnosis to keep me on track. I now embrace my new identity as a person both with bipolar and with many gifts and talents.

> "If I weren't bipolar, I wouldn't be me!"
> ~Colman-Hayes (2010:41)

I simply have to balance things to stay stable.

> "I fought hard for my health. And I won." ~McPheron (2010:52)

In 2011, I reflected in my journal:

> In a fundamental way
> My life is divided into two parts:
> before bipolar, and after.
>
> I spent years hankering for my "old life,"
> But now I realize that was not ideal in any way.
>
> Now I appreciate my "new life" –
> all the things I do to stay healthy.
>
> And all the things I never would've done
> without bipolar.
>
> I commit to continuing my healing.
>
> I will love and take care of myself.

"War stories" revisited

In the *Introduction,* I remembered my days as a nurse doing psych rotations. I mentioned some of the "war stories" I gathered from those experiences. I never imagined that one day I would become the protagonist in such stories.

What goes around comes around.

What might a teenaged student nurse make of some of my behaviours before, during and after hospitalization? What tales would she tell about this mad woman bolting from the house in mid-winter with no coat on, crawling down hospital corridors in the middle of the night, and frantically scribbling post-it notes to capture racing ideas for a book she was going to write one day.

"A book? Yeah, right!"

Yeah. Right!

A new perspective

Even though I trained as a nurse, and did those psych rotations, I was as prejudiced as the next person about mental illness. I felt an almost visceral discomfort about it, had no real understanding of it, and never questioned the stigmatization of people with mental illness.

Deep down, in some unexamined recess of my mind, I secretly blamed the victims for their illnesses, and felt oh-so-superior to them, being mentally sound and unmarred at the time.

How the mighty have fallen.

I now have nothing but empathy for all who are "mad like me" and I identify closely with their struggles and sufferings. I want to be part of the growing movement to dispel the stigma associated with mental illness, and hope that shining a light on my experiences with bipolar will help.

It's not only my personal experience with bipolar that's helped me gain a new perspective on mental illness, but all the reading and learning I have done since being diagnosed.

The books, journals, blogs and articles I have read, the coun-selling sessions and consultations with my psychiatrists over the years, the various psycho-education and mindfulness-based cognitive therapy courses I have done – all these have helped me gain a deeper understanding of mental illness.

What amazes me is how relatively little we still know about the brain and brain functioning. Consider that Dr. John Cade, an Australian psychiatrist, only discovered the therapeutic use of lithium by chance, in 1948.

He said: "I believe the brain, like any other organ, can get sick and it can also heal."

Encouraging words, but we still have a long way to go…

Reflections on writing this book

At a routine follow-up appointment several years ago now, Dr. R asked me what writing this book means to me. I said I was finding it therapeutic to look back on the process, and to make sense of what I – and my poor family – had been through.

While I was living through it, I felt like a victim of a massive flood, being swept downstream and never knowing when the next rapids or waterfall would hit. But by writing about it all, I was able to gain perspective. I was now in a helicopter looking down on that seething flood from a safe distance.

When Rob first read the manuscript, he said: "Wow; what an amazing accomplishment that you can write a book like you used to do before – despite bipolar and because of it."

I guess he's right. I do feel really good that it's done.

Make a quilt

It's been a potholed road with many, many episodes and two hospitalizations, but now that I have been stable for so long, I can reclaim aspects of my tattered life. I'm using the remnants to make a beautiful quilt.

May your quilt be both spectacular and comforting.

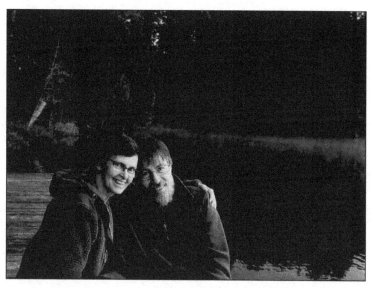

A quiet moment during a family vacation with all five kids, June 2017.

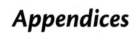

Appendices

Appendix 1: Definitions

History of bipolar disorder

> "Since antiquity, mood disorders have been recognized as biological illnesses that tend to run in families. Hippocrates [born in about 460 BC] described *melancholia*, or depression [...] Other Greek physicians saw in some people the tendency to change from the state of depression or melancholia into the agitated state of mania [...]"
> ~Benaur (2010:xviii)

Bipolar disorder used to be called "manic depression." In 1980, with the publication of the third edition of the *Diagnostic and Statistical Manual of Mental Disorders* (DSM-III), the name was officially changed to bipolar disorder.

Types of bipolar

> [Bipolar Type I and Bipolar Type II are the commonest forms, but] "we now also recognize that there are less severe forms of the illness that can be described [...] as *bipolar spectrum disorders*." ~Benaur (2010:xviii)

Bipolar I involves periods of depression and full-blown mania (defined below); Bipolar II involves depression and hypomania (also defined below).

Rapid cycling bipolar involves four or more episodes of depression and/or (hypo)mania per year.

Mania

Mania is a period of abnormally and persistently elevated, expansive or irritable mood and abnormally and persistently increased activity or energy lasting at least one week (or less if hospitalization is necessary) and including three or more of the following: elevated, expansive mood; inflated self-esteem or grandiosity; decreased need for sleep; more talkative than usual or pressure to keep talking; flight of ideas or racing thoughts; distractibility; increase in energy, goal-directed activity or psychomotor agitation; excessive involvement in pleasurable activities that have a high potential for painful consequences (e.g. spending sprees, foolish investments, speeding, drunk driving, risky sexual encounters). May be accompanied by psychosis (e.g. hallucinations, delusions).

Hypomania

Hypomania is a milder form of mania, lasting for at least four days, and not severe enough to warrant hospitalization or cause marked impairment in social or work functioning. There are no associated psychotic symptoms. All the other symptoms of mania apply, but in milder form. Untreated, a hypomanic episode can last anywhere from a few days to years; normally from a few weeks to months.

Depression

A major depressive episode is characterized by a severely depressed mood that lasts at least two weeks. (It may persist for many months if untreated.) Depressive episodes are classified as mild, moderate and severe depending on their impact on social or work functioning.

Symptoms of depression include: depressed mood (dysphoria); diminished interest or pleasure in activities; psychomotor retardation nearly every day (observable by others, not merely subjective feelings of being slowed down); fatigue or loss of energy; feelings of worthlessness or excessive or inappropriate guilt (not merely self-reproach or guilt about being ill); recurrent thoughts of death (not just fear of dying); recurrent suicidal ideation or a suicide attempt.

A person who has experienced depression and then has an episode of mania or hypomania is automatically given a diagnosis of bipolar disorder.

Episodes "with mixed features"

In the fifth and latest edition of the *Diagnostic and Statistical Manual of Mental Disorders* (DSM-V, 2013), there is a new emphasis on (hypo)manic and depressive episodes "with mixed features." This means that while the major features of the episode may be manic, there are three or more concurrent features of depression, and vice versa for depressive episodes with three or more features of mania or hypomania.

About 40% of bipolar patients experience episodes with mixed features at some point. Mixed depressive states are particularly dangerous: they are associated with more severe episodes, poorer prognosis and higher rates of concurrent illness. The three key symptoms of agitation, anxiety and irritability are significantly more common in bipolar depressive episodes with mixed features than in cases of major depressive disorder. Bipolar patients with these symptoms during a depressive episode need urgent help.

Epidemiology of bipolar disorder

> "[T]he estimated lifetime prevalence rate of [bipolar disorder] in Canada is 2.2%. This translates to well over 500,000 Canadians who would meet study criteria for mania at some point in their lives."
> ~Schaffer et al. (2006:13)

> "Bipolar I disorder affects approximately 1–2% of the population in the United States. Its usual onset is in later adolescence or young adulthood." ~Benaur (2010:xviii)

> "[Rapid cycling bipolar disorder] is rare, only seen in about 10% of patients with bipolar disorder, and for reasons that are still unclear seems to predominantly affect women." ~Benaur (2010:xxi)

How patients and family members experience bipolar

> "I felt like three little girls lived inside of me, one tired and sad, one too full of energy, always doing outrageous things, and the one who used to be me."
> ~Livesay (2010:45–46)

> "… [E]motions may be too intense, or there may be a lack of feelings that are appropriate to the situation. Moods may change too rapidly or not at all despite the occurrence of significant life events." ~Benaur (2010:xvii)

> "…[W]hen Joy [his wife] is calm – her normal self – the Other is lurking just beneath the surface of her eyes, examining me for the slightest hint that can be interpreted as an attack." ~Gore (2010:118)

Treatment

The main treatment for bipolar disorder is the mood stabilizer, lithium. Many patients may also need additional medications to achieve stability: anti-convulsants, anti-psychotics, anti-depressants, anti-anxiety medications and sedatives can be added in various combinations.

Prognosis

"Having successfully overcome the initial challenges of aberrant mood states, people [with bipolar] can and do lead emotionally rich and varied lives."
~Benaur (2010:xxvi)

So there is hope, then!

Appendix 2: Daily self-care chart and journal

"I have the writing demon that keeps my soul uplifted from deep darkness. Writing is my shield against madness. Writing keeps me sane!" ~O'Neal (2010:145)

The best way I know to learn about how bipolar affects you – and how you can affect bipolar! – is to keep a detailed daily chart and journal.

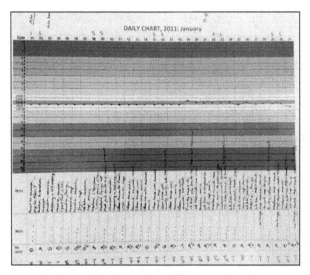

Sample of my daily chart during a period of stability in 2011.

I used a colourful chart, meant to clearly indicate lows (blues and greys) and highs (oranges and reds) deviating from the central green line that indicates normal mood. Later, I realized that I was wasting a lot of expensive ink and settled for a chart with a single green line in the centre.

Your doctor may have given you a daily chart, or you could design your own one, as I did. I created columns for each day of the month, and rows to chart my mood (−10 for the deepest depression, 0 for normal mood, and +10 for the highest mania), activities I did that day (e.g. meditation, exercise, total hours of work, etc.), meds taken (I just use ditto marks if nothing has changed in my meds regime), hours of sleep, and minutes or hours spent napping during the day.

Occasionally, I would ask Rob to rate my mood on the same scale I was using, just to get his perspective. Interestingly, when I was depressed or stable, there was no difference between our ratings. But when I was becoming (hypo)manic, he would often rate me higher than I did, assessing me as more (hypo)manic than I did. This irritated me: I felt judged and patronized by his *tsk-tsk* assessments. I thought I was doing rather well keeping it all together and wanted recognition for that.

I desperately needed his approval when I was "off." I guess I felt understandably vulnerable.

Looking back, he was probably quite correct. My judgments − even of my own mood and behaviour − surely got clouded by the (hypo)mania itself.

I keep my journal on the back side of the chart and make a note of anything significant that happened during the day or any mood swings.

These are some excerpts from my April 2009 journal:

1. *[Emerging from depression:]* Feeling great − optimistic, planning travel for summer! Joy − to be "back"!

2. *[Next day:]* I'm back! Great day.

3. *[Next day:]* ?Slightly hypomanic. Lots of travel plans! Smiling all day!

4. *[Two days later:]* A bit hypomanic at Cooper's Marsh: running around chasing a poor goose! But it was funny; not too weird or uncharacteristic, I don't think. Great day! Big smiles!

5. *[Four days later:]* Definite hypomanic "spike" – felt "fizzing"! "Creative storm" and flight of ideas. Only got 1.5 hours of sleep. Busy-busy with all kinds of creative projects and plans, but zero work-work done. Poor Rob soldiered on alone.

6. *[Three days later:]* Expansive hypomanic spike continues. I am 100% happy and joyful, but Rob gets very ratty and rude with me. He finds me pushy, demanding and bossy, and says he has to dig in and assert himself. I say, "But I'm SICK! How come you're so caring when I go down, but such a jerk when I'm up?!" Huge fight in the bedroom at 2:30 a.m. – I went downstairs to cool off and get away from him. Awful night. Total of 4 hours sleep in 4 short sessions.

7. *[Seven days later:]* Felt a bit off today. Woke up feeling sluggish and didn't want to get out of bed. Please don't tell me this is another depression starting...

After some months or even years of daily charting (sure, it takes commitment, but do you want to take control of your bipolar or not?), you can eventually discern patterns. Ask yourself:

1. What triggers my depressions? (Did I forget my meds the day before? Did I not get enough sleep? Did I argue with someone?)

2. Do I have more depressions than (hypo)manias?

3. How long does each episode last?

4. Do I get a period of normal mood in be-
    tween episodes?

5. Do I have rapid cycling bipolar (four or
    more episodes per year)?

And so on. And once you know more about how the disorder
affects you from day-to-day and week-to-week, you will be
better able to control it.

I also recommend keeping close track of the self-care
strategies you use to keep bipolar under control. Every evening, check off on a table: did I take my meds as prescribed;
exercise; eat a balanced diet; sleep enough last night; have
some social contact; relax; laugh; avoid caffeine, alcohol and
drugs; meditate; use other stress reduction techniques; etc.
Aim for 10/10 eventually but do start somewhere and build
up.

The basic idea is to structure your life in such a way that
bipolar can't gain a foothold. Tracking your strategies by
charting every day keeps your recovery program clearly in
your mind. If you let the charting slip, I can almost guarantee
that your commitment to your recovery will soon slip as well.

Good records will also keep your care provider fully informed about what has been happening to you since your last
appointment.

> "I began charting my moods and finding small things
> that affected how I felt. I began to analyze situations
> that led to rage and tried to learn how I could regain
> control. In doing so, I improved my self-esteem and I
> started to feel like I had some control over my life
> again." ~Pilkington (2010:171)

Appendix 3: Self-care for stability

Table of Contents for Appendix 3

Introduction

I want to be perfectly clear: I am no paragon of virtue. The strategies that I believe help me stay stable are by no means always faithfully applied. I often scold myself for slacking off in one area or another: I can always do better. I urge you to make a start and do whatever seems useful to you to help bring your own bipolar under control. If what works for me can help you in any way, I'll be delighted. If it stimulates you to think of other strategies that better suit your needs and preferences, so much the better. Either way, know that you are human and will, in all likelihood, slip up from time to time.

Just as I do.

Having said that, though, let's face facts: this is a very, very serious disorder we are battling, so it deserves careful and concerted attention. It's simply not good enough to have an "I'll do it when I feel like it" attitude towards your self-care program. If that's the best you can do, bipolar will surely win.

1. Get a diagnosis

> "Ten years [is] approximately the [...] length of time it takes for someone with bipolar disorder to receive a proper diagnosis." ~Garey (2010:xxvii)

Maybe you recognize some of the moods and behaviours described in this book but have never been diagnosed as having bipolar. Maybe you think you have depression. Anxiety. A personality disorder. Or maybe nothing at all. I cannot urge you strongly enough to get assessed and get a proper diagnosis so you can then get appropriate treatment. Untreated, bipolar episodes tend to get worse and worse, as the brain hardwires itself for the extreme ups and downs, rather than for normal moods.

2. Accept the diagnosis

> "I am a person with a mental illness. So it takes some extra effort. So sometimes it's debilitating. But now that I'm learning to manage it, it's becoming not my entire life but simply a part of how I live, something the people around me live with as well, something I can accept. I have to. That's the only way this works." ~Hornbacher (2008:214)

Once you are diagnosed, get a second opinion if you feel that's needed, but then don't waste time – like I did – before accepting the diagnosis. Don't play the denial game, or the blame-the-doctor game, or any other game that's going to prevent you from staring bipolar in the evil eye and saying: "OK, I have bipolar. That really sucks. Now what?"

3. Accept the seriousness of the disorder

Accept that you have a disorder that will most likely need life-long treatment, and one that has a very high rate of suicide associated with it. About 10–20% of bipolar patients die by suicide, and according to Jamison (2000), at least 25–50% of bipolar patients attempt suicide at least once. Those are truly shocking statistics.

Don't mess with bipolar: treat it with the utmost respect.

4. Learn as much as possible about the disorder

a. Psycho-education

Some hospitals and community clinics offer psycho-education courses to inform bipolar patients (and their carers) about the disorder, treatment options, and self-care strategies. Ask around until you find a course you can attend. It's not only invaluable to learn the information, but it's great to spend time with fellow bipolar patients and to compare notes with them.

I attended two psycho-education courses – one at the Douglas and one at a community clinic. For the first course, I was still mentally foggy from my high doses of meds and couldn't participate optimally. For the second course a year later, I was able to stay focused throughout the sessions. I asked questions, made suggestions, and did my homework faithfully. I felt like a real student again. It was a liberation. The old academic in me was surfacing once more, raising her beaten and bruised head tentatively to see if this newfound clarity was real or only imagined. Each week, I approached the session with some trepidation in case I lost focus again. Thankfully, I completed the 18-week course with no problems.

b. Reading

Read all the resources provided in your psycho-education course; read books about bipolar from the library, that you order online or buy at the bookstore; and read articles and blogs on the Internet. Read about the disorder itself, about treatment options, about medications, and about side effects. Read personal accounts written by people with bipolar. You want as much information as possible, so you can face your dragon well-armed. And so that you can ask relevant questions of your care provider.

Don't feel bad if you can't make it through a whole section or chapter at one time. That will improve as your brain heals. Maybe start with smaller sessions online where the information is presented in bite-sized pieces. Or just read a couple of paragraphs at a time. Just get those neurons firing again!

There's a list of references and resources at the end of this book to get you started.

c. Therapy

You will remember the empathetic counsellor Rob and I saw at Friends for Mental Health, Lucy Lu. We both learned an enormous amount about bipolar and how to deal with it from her. I wish every family had access to such quality care. Try to find a therapist to teach you coping strategies, and who you can relate to.

5. Accept treatment

After all your learning and reading, the moment of truth comes. Are you going to accept psychiatric medications, or do you want to consult one or more alternative healers (e.g. acupuncturist, naturopath, homeopath, etc.)? I delayed accepting the medications by a few months while I used acupuncture and naturopathy instead. It was only when I dropped into a second bleak depression that I relented and accepted lithium treatment. Since then, other medications have been added and subtracted as my psychiatrists struggled to find just the right combinations and dosages for me. Overall, I have no regrets about accepting the meds.

Whatever you decide for your own treatment plan, do accept treatment of some kind. Bipolar is not going to control itself.

a. Medications

If you decide to use mainstream psychiatric medications, as I eventually did, remember that meds can only help manage, not cure, bipolar.

> "Medical science has no cure for bipolar disorder, but it does have an arsenal with which to combat the symptoms." ~D'Ascoli (2010:79)

Don't-don't-don't stop taking your meds once you feel better: you'll land (back) in the hospital. If you stop your meds, your bipolar episodes may recur even worse than before.

> "I never forget to take my meds. They are my food, water and sunshine." ~Rusczyk (2010:15)

I swallow my meds religiously. I have a chart right beside the pill bottles next to my toothbrush, and I mark off every time I swallow a pill so I never forget to take a dose. (Ask your pharmacist what to do if you miss a dose by mistake.) I know exactly what is at stake if my blood levels get too low, and I have been there, done that, thank you.

I don't stop my meds when I feel well; and I don't reduce the dose because of side effects. I do discuss my concerns with my psychiatrist, and she does whatever she feels is safe to reduce the doses when possible. But she is still watching me like a hawk after the two hospitalization incidents over eight years ago now.

> "Lamictal [an anti-convulsant used to treat both epilepsy and bipolar] saved my sanity. Yes, I hate being dependent on medication. Yes, I hate being put in the category of the mentally ill... But I have my family back, can set my priorities more intelligently, and [...] focus on myself and my health for the first time in my life. Today, I am a highly functional adult with bipolar disorder who can identify triggers and avoid self-destructive behavior with a little help from my friend, Lamictal." ~Norman (2010:63)

b. Accept the effects of medications

The biggest effect that you might notice when your meds kick in is the lack of (hypo)manic highs: those "wonderful" periods of grandiosity, energy and elation when you were on top of the world and felt you could do anything you wanted. To be perfectly frank, I miss those times now. I feel flattened out, somewhat dumbed down, rather boring. I know there is that other reality just behind the veil of normalcy, but I dare not lift the curtain again. I might be swept off-stage forever.

If you need to mourn your hypomanic episodes, go right ahead and mourn. But always keep your eye on the ultimate goal: stability.

Equally noticeable, I hope, will be the lack of depressive holes in your life. This has been the biggest gift the meds have given me, and I am so thankful.

Even though the gift sometimes comes with a price: side effects.

c. Accept the side effects of medications

"The laundry list of meds he had prescribed left her exhausted and sleeping 17 hours a day, and for the few hours she was awake, she was sullen and unemotional." ~McKinstry (2010:114)

"My latest medication has turned me into a ravenous foodaholic…" ~Rowe (2010:21)

I now accept the side effects of my meds. Lord knows, I'd love not to have a weight problem, hand tremors, skin rashes, a need for countless extra hours of sleep each week, excessive thirst, frequent urination, thinning bones, and so on. But all these things are simply side effects of meds I know I need (or needed at the time). Each person reacts differently to the meds, and these just happened to be the side effects that I got. When I compare them to the alternative – relentless rapid cycling bipolar episodes – there is no doubt in my mind that the side effects were a very small price to pay. At least I could

function with them, whereas before, I was completely paralyzed when depressed, or running rabid when (hypo)manic.

As my disorder has been reined in, and my meds adjusted and doses reduced, my side effects have diminished
markedly. Today, shaky hands, thirst, frequent urination, and
the need to sleep a bit more than I used to are my main com-
plaints.

Small price to pay.

6.   Build a healthy lifestyle

We must accept that there are things we ourselves can do to
help control bipolar. There's no guarantee, and there will be
many slips along the way, but self-care is a critical part of the
whole picture. Just as a diabetic must comply with dietary restrictions as well as take insulin, so we bipolar sufferers have
to take responsibility for learning about how the disorder affects us personally, and for building a healthy lifestyle that will
minimize our chances of triggering a bipolar episode and
maximize our chances of maintaining a normal mood.

Different people will find different strategies more helpful in building a healthy lifestyle, but this is what works for
me.

a.   Get good sleep

> "Protecting sleep and developing a more organized
> lifestyle can be as valuable in maintaining recovery as
> medications." ~Benaur (2010:xxv)

I go to bed at more-or-less the same time every night and
wake up at more-or-less the same time every morning. Even
on weekends. I'm rigorously disciplined about this. I need

more sleep than the average adult thanks to my meds. Even for special occasions like birthdays or weddings, I don't extend my normal bedtime beyond an hour or two maximum, and then I either sleep in or nap the next day. This consistency of sleep really helps me to avoid getting over-excited and therefore at risk of hypomania, or over-tired and at risk of depression. Lack of sleep – even being just an hour or two short of what your body and brain needs – is a major trigger for many people. Please monitor yourself.

When I was (hypo)manic, I was prescribed Zopiclone, a sleeping pill to take on an "as needed" basis. It slowed me down enough to get at least some sleep when I could easily have stayed up buzzing all night. Nowadays, I use Zopiclone on very rare occasions – maybe once every two or three months – when I can feel a bubbly, excited feeling in my belly at bedtime, and I know that sleep is going to be slow in coming.

I am as protective of my time with sleep as I would be with a lover. Every moment together is precious and must be jealously guarded against the distractions that would separate us every night: Netflix, news magazines, books, the heat pump clunking on and off, a distant train at 4 a.m., and of course, my bladder. All these must be resisted, ignored, or if I have to respond, put out of mind as quickly and calmly as possible, so I don't fully waken and lose skin contact with my sleep-lover.

b. Meditate daily

I meditate for fifteen to twenty minutes a day. I learned about meditation in two different groups in the community, and in a mindfulness-based cognitive therapy (MBCT) group at the

Douglas Hospital. There are countless excellent guided meditation apps and sessions on YouTube – experiment until you find voices, accents, music and visuals you like.

Taking this time to calm and centre myself really helps to slow me down. It also reminds me of the importance of taking care of myself, every day. When I am in the rocking chair with the headphones plugged in, it alerts the family that I am nurturing myself, and thus keeps my disorder on the agenda in a positive way: she's making an effort to stay well. I hope it also teaches them something about persistence and dedication to a program.

c. Reduce stress

As I see it, there are two ways to reduce stress: circumstantially and attitudinally. Avoid stressful *circumstances* that you know will affect you negatively: heavy traffic, visits to toxic relatives, confrontations with your boss, whatever. However, if you can't avoid these circumstances for whatever reason, use your mental powers to change your *attitude* towards the situation. For example, consider that traffic gives time to enjoy classical music or catch up on world events on the car radio. Dinner with negative relatives gives you a chance to do quiet deep breathing as their rude comments flow over you like water off a proverbial duck's back. And so on.

I try to leave five minutes early every time I go out. And I sometimes deliberately move over from the fast to the slow lane on the highway, and enjoy mindfully, contentedly travelling at a slower pace – I give myself some breathing space.

Speaking of breathing, I use the little calming exercise of taking three deep, cleansing breaths at any time during the day when I feel stress building up, or when I have to wait. For example, YouTube sometimes takes a moment to load, so I breathe deeply. Time passes faster, and I calm myself at the same time.

I use music to relax me as well. When I'm driving, I often switch from talk radio to classical music. Calm music helps relax me; cheery music (upbeat, fast-paced, or songs I can sing along to) helps when I feel a bit down.

I need much more "alone time" nowadays. For example, I like to eat breakfast when there is no one else in the kitchen. No interactions, no expectations, no stress. I've told Rob not to take this distancing personally. It just seems that my brain still needs downtime during the day to function well. And I know better than to talk back to my temperamental brain.

d. Avoid alcohol and drugs

> "Most psychiatrists and psychologists agree that if you have bipolar disorder, you should avoid alcohol and recreational drugs altogether." ~Miklowitz (2002:174)

As a Baha'i, I don't use either alcohol or recreational drugs, so this is not an issue for me. But for many bipolar sufferers, substance use can be a huge factor. According to the website http://bipolar.about.com, 30–60% of people with bipolar disorder also struggle with alcoholism or substance abuse, perhaps in an attempt to self-medicate.

Drugs and alcohol are dangerous in bipolar disorder. Just think: these are mind-altering substances that we then introduce into our already fragile, unstable, and prescription-medicated minds. Is that not asking for trouble?

After the buzz of being high or drunk, people come down, and this can trigger a depressed state. Playing with fire. As well, many have a hard time drinking in moderation; they get out of control and then become destabilized.

Does any of this sound familiar to you? If so, ask yourself an ultra-serious question: do you want the best chance of controlling your disorder, or do you want to continue using alcohol and/or other substances, putting your mental health at severe risk? Actually, not only your mental health, but your entire life: substance use is associated with a much higher risk of suicide in bipolar patients (Jamison, 2000).

Depending on how far you have already gone down the road, you may need to seek professional counselling for drug or alcohol addiction. If so, please don't delay. Your stability – your life – is on the line.

e. Don't over-work

I used to be a workaholic, slaving away at either volunteer or paid work for fifteen or more hours a day, even while raising a young family. That has had to stop, for two reasons. First, the meds simply don't allow me the kind of awake time I'd need to keep up that pace. But second, I have made a conscious commitment to reform myself. Except in exceptional circumstances and for short bursts of time, I don't hope to work more than eight hours a day anymore. That leaves me time for daily meditation, regular exercise, and relaxation. I complete a decent amount of work and feel much more balanced than I used to.

f. Eat healthy food

Eating a healthy diet is a key part of taking care of myself. I try to eat at regular times each day and we often eat vegetarian food. I limit sugar intake and only drink decaf coffee to avoid over-stimulation of my brain. (Caffeine is, after all, a stimulant that alters the functioning of our brains.) It's all just part of regulating my entire life and taking the best possible care of myself.

g. Exercise regularly

I exercise in our well-equipped basement gym at least three times a week, sometimes four or five times. At first, Karrie and Tami were my exercise buddies, keeping me on track. Then, Rob and I exercised together. Just recently, I hired a personal trainer who comes to our home twice a week to supervise my workouts. (I'm hoping not only to get fitter and stronger, but also to prevent further loss of bone density, which is a side effect of Epival.)

I also joined weekly Tai Chi and Zumba classes for several years, and more recently, clog dancing. I really enjoy getting out and being with a group of people for these classes.

For depression prevention, you can't beat regular exercise. Brisk walks. Karate. Ballet. Hockey. Yoga. Tennis. Whatever works for you. As the ad says: "Just do it."

h. Maintain social contact

Maintaining social contact is an important part of staying in balance. I totally withdrew from my social network when I was depressed and tended to get over-excited by social contact when I went up. Now that I am in a normal mood, I try to structure social time every week: over the years since I was diagnosed, I've attended a bipolar support group, French lessons, a Creative Journaling course, joined Toastmasters, a book club, and an improv group. In addition, I have several Baha'i-related responsibilities: administrative meetings, devotional gatherings, study groups. All these commitments get me out of the house and provide both social and intellectual stimulation.

i.   Seek intellectual stimulation

My brain atrophied during all the months of mental inactivity throughout the ups and downs of untreated or inadequately treated rapid cycling bipolar. Then there were the meds that made me feel foggy, amnesiac and incapable of intellectual accomplishment. I was dumbed down, and needed to relearn how to think clearly, creatively and sharply.

Practice makes perfect. I started with small steps, doing crossword puzzles and Sudoku, then trying to read short articles in a news magazine. Often, I couldn't focus to the end. Later on, I got better, and actually enjoyed reading again. Then I tackled articles in professional journals. At first, I had to complete an article in several small sittings. Gradually, I could read more than a few complex paragraphs at a time. Now, I can swallow the whole beast in one big gulp. Even hundred-page reports don't intimidate me in the least.

Same goes for writing. At first, drafting even a simple email felt overwhelming. Now, I can write long reports, training manuals, and... well... this book.

j.   Cultivate hobbies

This is one area I would like to do better in. I can't really call meditation or daily exercise "hobbies," after all. I spend a lot of evening time watching Netflix. It's relaxing, and I love do-ing it, but does that qualify? It's such a passive pastime… I do enjoy reading and play a bit of piano and guitar. It's good exercise for the brain at the same time as being good for the soul.

Having a hobby is part of living a balanced life. Find something you enjoy doing that helps you slow down and feel relaxed while also giving you a sense of accomplishment.

k. Be assertive

If you're going to stay on track, week in, week out, month in, month out, you need to be your own best advocate. You can't allow others to put your stability at risk. "Shall we watch a movie tonight?" No, thanks; I'm going to the gym for my ex-ercise session. "How about a drink after work?" No, thanks; I don't drink anymore. "Want to go clubbing with the gang?" No, thanks; I need to be in bed at a reasonable hour.

Worried that "no" appears too often? Just remember that at the same time, you are saying "no" to dreadful epi-sodes of depression and (hypo)mania. Saying "no" to risky be-haviour means saying "yes" to your precious mental health.

You might try offering alternative activities that won't jeopardize your stability. Movie night? "Sure, but let's start early so I can get to sleep on time." Drinks after work? "Sure, but I'll stick to non-alcoholic drinks," or "How about meeting at a coffee shop instead?" And so on.

l. Develop a positive attitude

"[…] I thought to myself: I have to be able to change my thoughts, to distract myself, not by drugs or drink but by positive actions. I had been given the tools to

> do so. I have a choice – to switch from negative
> thoughts to positive ones, to make the light reappear
> and the darkness recede." ~Trudeau (2010: 306)

Many people habitually think negatively. It's their default position. Life sucks. I'll never be well again. Why me? And so on, endlessly. No wonder these people are miserable; they make themselves so.

Try switching the voice in your head. Life is beautiful and amazing; I am so happy to be alive. I'm on the path to wellness. I am taking control of my life. I'm lucky to have such caring friends and relatives.

> "Having bipolar disorder is very difficult, but I'm
> proud that I've learned to manage it by facing it. I now
> understand that even if I get a negative thought or
> emotion, I can take a step back and realize that it's not
> going to overtake me or control me." ~Stearn
> (2010:159)

Just try meditating about what makes you joyful and grateful. I guarantee that if you do that for one minute today, tomorrow you'll want to do it for two minutes – or more. It grows on you. It becomes a new way of being. And slowly, your frown and down-turned mouth will soften; you'll start to smile again.

In *The Secret* (2006), Rhonda Byrne advises us to make a list of all the wonderful and funny things that have happened in our lives, so we can refer to it when we feel negative. I find this especially useful when I really relive those past experiences in detail, remembering the sounds, sights, smells, tastes and other sensory feelings as well as the emotions. I can't help but smile at some of the events. And one smile soon leads to another.

Fast & Preston (2004) advise us to act "as if": when depressed, we should act *as if* things are better than they are. We can then fool the brain into feeling better. And when all else fails, remember the old AA motto: "One day at a time." Things will eventually improve; for now, just get through today.

m. Use your body to fool your brain!

Use your body to trick your mind. For example, studies have shown that simply standing up from a lying or seated position makes people feel stronger and more optimistic. Walking over to a window and gazing out is even better. Or step outside and look up at the sky. Just the act of getting the fluid swirling in your inner ear helps lift your mood. Swinging, rocking, rolling down a hill, brisk walking or jogging has the same effect: all these activities get that fluid circulating.

Use "power poses" to boost your confidence: stand with feet shoulder-width apart, arms raised high overhead or spread out wide, fingers stretched wide, chest puffed out proudly and head thrown back. Pretend you just won an Olympic sprint! Now, take three slow, deep breaths in that position, and smile widely. You'll feel like a winner!

And even if you can't crack a smile – which lifts your mood automatically, by the way – just hold a pencil lengthwise between your teeth: your "smile muscles" will automatically be activated, and your brain will be fooled into thinking you're having a great day!

n. Get support

If you can possibly arrange it, ask a spouse, sibling, parent or friend to offer you support and motivate you to stay on track with medications, medical visits and lifestyle changes.

A note to loved ones & carers about your own lifestyle

If you're reading this book because someone you know has bipolar disorder, please pause and ask yourself: What can I *myself* do to build a healthy lifestyle to stay mentally healthy?

Please don't take your own mental health for granted or put it at risk while you focus too much on your loved one. If you burn out and crash, there may be no one to take care of either of you!

7.   Other steps to keep bipolar in check

Apart from taking your medications (or alternative treatments) faithfully and living a healthy lifestyle, what else can you do to help keep bipolar in check?

a. Learn about your triggers

Triggers are things (people, events, emotions, circumstances, places, etc.) that cause bipolar symptoms. Why is it so important to learn about your triggers? Because if you don't, the leaky faucet will keep spilling water all over the floor, and your family and friends will be left to mop up the mess. But if you do, you can literally turn off the tap and stop the flood at its source.

So, look at bipolar symptoms as a clue, and ask yourself: what might have caused these symptoms at this time? A common trigger is stress: this may be negative stress like work- or school-related deadlines, fights with family members, death of a loved one, etc.; or positive stress like social events, travel, marriage, birth of a baby, etc. Other triggers include alcohol or drug use, lack of sleep, and so on.

What are your personal triggers for both depression and (hypo)mania?

When I looked back at my whole history with bipolar, studying my daily charts and all the notes I had made, I could identify triggers or potential triggers for about 80% of all my episodes. In the other 20% of cases, my mood simply switched, unannounced, apparently of its own accord. Infuriating when you're focused on prevention. In my case, then, trigger-analysis was not foolproof, but it was a great help.

From the analysis I did, I learned that triggers for depression included my emotional reaction to a family drama in which I had become emotionally over-involved, getting sick with a bad cold, feeling uncomfortable in a social situation, attending a wedding, and a work-related deadline. Triggers for (hypo)mania included going on vacation, seasonal change (springtime), lack of sleep, stress around the time of my mom's death, and starting on Epival (that was ironic!). There were also a few cases where I could identify triggers that pulled me back from depression and brought me into normal mood: work-related travel (three times), a trip to a cottage with all five children present, and starting on Seroquel.

When family dramas inevitably arise, I am now armed with my daily guided meditation practice and my "meditation frame of mind" to protect me from getting overheated emotionally. Because a bout of sickness triggered a depression, I now get flu shots every year. (I never used to do so.) If I ever end up in a situation that makes me feel uncomfortable for any reason, I will assert myself and leave at once. I don't have to account to anyone for my "rude" behaviour: there's way too much at stake. This includes leaving parties and weddings early if the noise and stimulation feels too much for me. Work-related deadlines are often negotiable. I am now rigid about bedtime every night. I have to protect my brain by getting enough sleep, consistently. Finally, God forbid if I get depressed again, I will ask Rob to take me to the mountains or a lake for a day trip or short retreat, hoping that the time away will reverse whatever weird chemical reaction has triggered the depression.

b. Learn to identify your early warning signs

Once something (or nothing you can identify!) has triggered an episode, the idea is to recognize your early warning signs as soon as possible to prevent a full-blown episode. Different people have different warning signs, but we can all learn to detect our signs and figure out strategies to prevent early signs from snowballing. Recall the accounts in Chapter 15 of how I used early warning signs to head off hypomanic and depressive blips that threatened to engulf me.

I have analyzed my own episodes, using my daily charts, notes and memories. Some of the key warning signs of depression include "the veil" that comes down around my head; lack of energy; a leaden feeling in my limbs; emotional distance from my family and friends; inability to focus; failure to check emails regularly; and lack of interest in things I normally care about. I now know to go into major attack mode to keep a severe depression at bay. Exercise, regular sleep (but not too much sleep), good food, doing fun activities, and as many of the things I discussed in Section 6 above ("Build a healthy lifestyle") as I can manage.

For (hypo)mania, one of my earliest warning signs is a bubbly, excited feeling in my stomach. I get an interest (totally uncharacteristic) in interior design and beautification projects. I become more outgoing and social and also enjoy spending money more than usual. Thoughts about how nice it would be to visit a spa again come back to me: for long months in between, spas have seemed frivolous and exorbitant. In the same way, I make hopeful travel plans to exotic destinations: China, Cuba, Jamaica, Hawaii, wherever. Bring it on! Flashes of irritability – mainly reserved for Rob, poor soul – is also a key sign. As well, I want to stay up way past my normal bedtime, feeling full of energy and brimming with great ideas that need my attention right away.

Learn to recognize your own early warning signs for both (hypo)mania and depression. Write them down so you can refer to them when you start to go up or down. And learn to respond to them promptly with your full attention and intelligence so you can prevent a full-blown episode if that's at all possible.

c.   Create an action plan to prevent episodes

Having a list of early warning signs is a great first step. But you also need notes about what specific steps you can take to try to head off an episode. Then, as soon as you recognize the early signs of an impending (hypo)manic or depressive episode, you can implement a clear and simple *action plan* to try to curb it.

Write down your emergency plans (one for highs, one for lows) and file them safely so you can refer to them as soon as you identify a sudden spike or dip and feel the onset of those dreaded early warning signs.

Again, please refer to Chapter 15 where I describe specific actions I took to prevent both hypomanic and depressive blips from progressing to full-blown episodes.

Of course, there's no guarantee that your action plan will work every time, but it's well worth a try.

d. Learn how the disorder affects you

How does depression manifest in you? What negative thought patterns emerge? How can you nip these in the bud and change your thinking before the negativity becomes entrenched? How do you behave when (hypo)manic? Is irritability or anxiety a feature of your disorder? How does bipolar affect your relationships? Really stare down this beast and get to know it from the inside out. Only when you truly understand what you're up against can you devise effective strategies to cope with it.

As I said in Appendix 2, one of the best ways to get to know how bipolar affects you – and how you can affect your bipolar – is to keep a daily self-care chart and journal.

e. Accept the realities of the disorder

Part of coming to terms with your diagnosis is accepting the cyclical nature of the fiend. The ups and downs are, quite simply, what bipolar is all about. Don't rail against it; it is what it is, and your job is to figure out the best possible ways to control those highs and lows using every means you can.

When I first got sick, I wasted many months feeling sorry for myself and being angry at the universe. Not productive. Not healthy. But you know what? I won't beat myself up too badly about my immature and unspiritual initial response. We all deserve a little time for grieving when we're slapped with a diagnosis like this.

8. Accept the impact of bipolar on your family and friends

Bipolar is a family disorder: our moods and behaviours affect everyone around us. We must accept that.

> "If I'm not careful … Joy's [his wife's] illness will drive me insane, too. Take me right down with it. Then up. Then down again… The two-edged sword of caring for her while caring about her is already carving me up so badly." ~Gore (2010:120)

Bipolar can strain a relationship to the point of no return. Tread carefully.

> "During periods of stabilization, I focused on understanding how my illness impacted my family and friends. I realized that it was a struggle for them as well. Relationships are difficult for both sides and dealing with something as difficult as bipolar disorder can cause a great deal of resentment. My husband resented the fact that I was no longer the person he married. I resented him because he didn't understand what I was going through… I knew I had to try to make things easier for both of us to save our marriage. It motivated me to push harder." ~Pilkington (2010:170–171)

> "Who's crazy… / The one who sees doctors/ or the one who just waits in the car?" ~Yorkey (2010:17)

There's a great resource for couples called *Loving Someone with Bipolar Disorder* by Julie Fast (bipolar activist, columnist and administrator of www.bipolarhappens.com) and John Preston (clinical psychologist) that Rob found really helpful. When my head had cleared sufficiently for me to read a book, I delved into it to see what he had been learning. I found it interesting, practical and user-friendly, and I highly recommend it.

Some people are lucky enough to have a partner who stays loyal throughout:

> "[My husband] Don has been a real rock for me, though it's been hard for him sometimes. I once asked him why he didn't just leave and find someone else. His reply was, 'Don't worry about that, I'm not going anywhere. If you want to worry about something, worry about lightning striking.'" ~Friedlander (2010:164)

But we mustn't underestimate the stress of family members:

> "[Husband to wife with bipolar:] I know you're hurting. I am, too… I am the one who knows you,/ I am the one who cares,/ I am the one who's always been there./ I am the one who's helped you/ And if you think that I just don't give a damn,/ Then you just don't know who I am." ~Yorkey (2010:32–33)

9. Talk about your disorder with people you trust

Whether to disclose your diagnosis at all, and if so, to whom, is a deeply personal decision. It will depend on your circumstances and your own feelings of stigma about bipolar. There's a continuum from "keep it as secret as possible" on the left, to "disclose it to as many people as possible" on the right. You'll decide what feels right for you, but I do hope that you have at least a small circle of family and friends who understand, accept and love you and will support you through the inevitable ups and downs of your illness.

I have tended to be closer to the right-hand side of the continuum than the left: I find it therapeutic to tell people about what I have been through, and besides, I now consider mental illness to be no different than any other chronic illness like arthritis or diabetes. Another major advantage of personal disclosure is that each time one of us speaks out, we help to dispel the stigma of mental illness.

~   ~   ~

Fasten your seatbelt!

Consider this analogy. Getting a diagnosis and going on treatment is like installing a seatbelt for ourselves. But if we don't fasten that belt, it can do us no good. Using the self-care strategies outlined here is like clicking our seatbelt securely. There's no guarantee that we won't be in an accident, but at least we'll have that minimum protection.

We owe it to ourselves – and our families – to buckle up.

References and resources

Where relevant, I have updated this list with the latest editions of books that I originally used when I was first diagnosed.

Avrutis, V. "The Struggle and the Hope" pages 65–68 in Gore, RD & Garey, J. (eds.) (2010).

Basco, MR. (2015) *The Bipolar Workbook: Tools for Controlling Your Mood Swings.* 2nd edition. The Guilford Press, New York.

Benaur, M. "An Introduction to Bipolar Disorder" pages xvii–xxvi in Gore, RD & Garey, J. (eds.) (2010).

Byrne, R. (2006) *The Secret.* Atria Books, New York.

Caponigro, JM., Lee, EH., et al. (2012) *Bipolar Disorder: A Guide for the Newly Diagnosed.* New Harbinger Publications, Oakland, CA.

Colman-Hayes, S. "There's Always Something More Than Meets the Eye" pages 39–41 in Gore, RD & Garey, J. (eds.) (2010).

Cowan, G. (2013) *Back from the Brink: True Stories & Practical Help for Overcoming Depression & Bipolar Disorder.* New Harbinger Publications, Oakland, CA.

D'Ascoli, PF. "My Mother's Keeper" pages 77–79 in Gore, RD & Garey, J. (eds.) (2010).

Fast, JA. & Preston, J. (2006) *Take Charge of Bipolar Disorder: A 4-Step Plan for You and Your Loved Ones to Manage the Illness and Create Lasting Stability.* Wellness Central, New York.

Fast, JA. & Preston, JD. (2008) *Get It Done When You're Depressed: 50 Strategies for Keeping Your Life on Track.* Alpha Books, New York.

Fast, JA. & Preston, JD. (2011) *Loving someone with bipolar disorder: Understanding and helping your partner.* 2nd edition. New Harbinger Publications Inc., Oakland, CA.

Flynn, SC. "My Vision of Recovery" pages 69–74 in Gore, RD & Garey, J. (eds.) (2010).

Friedlander, B. "Dear Valerie" pages 161–167 in Gore, RD & Garey, J. (eds.) (2010).

Garey, J. "Next to Normal: Bipolar Disorder Takes Center Stage" pages xxvii–xxxvi in Gore, RD & Garey, J. (eds.) (2010).

Gore, RD. "Just a Normal Girl" pages 117–120 in Gore, RD & Garey, J. (eds.) (2010).

Gore, RD & Garey, J. for The Healing Project (eds.) (2010) *Voices of Bipolar Disorder – The healing companion: Stories for courage, comfort and strength.* Lachance Publishing, New York.

Greenberger, D. & Padesky, CA. (1995) *Mind Over Mood: Change How You Feel by Changing the Way You Think.* The Guilford Press, New York.

Hope, C. (2015) *Bipolar Disorder – The complete survival guide to stopping mood swings, and taking control of your life today!* Lean You LLC., New Jersey. (Kindle edition.)

Hornbacher, M. (2009) *Madness: A Bipolar Life.* Mariner Books, Boston.

Jameson, BR. (2012) *Transcending Bipolar Disorder: My Own True Story of Recovery from Mental Illness.* iUniverse Inc., Bloomington, IN.

Jamison, KR. (1996) *An Unquiet Mind: a memoir of moods and madness.* Vintage Books, New York.

Jamison, KR. "Suicide and bipolar disorder." *Journal of Clinical Psychiatry,* 2000;61 Supplement 9:47–51.

Kübler-Ross, E. (1969) *On Death and Dying: What the Dying Have to Teach Doctors, Nurses, Clergy, and their Own Families.* Touchstone, New York.

Livesay, G. "The Girl Who Used To Be Me" pages 45–48 in Gore, RD & Garey, J. (eds.) (2010).

Lowe, C. & Cohen, BM. (2010) *Living with Someone Who's Living with Bipolar Disorder.* Jossey-Bass, San Francisco.

McKinstry, J. "Husband's Two Cents" pages 113–116 in Gore, RD & Garey, J. (eds.) (2010).

McPheron, S. "A New Painting" pages 49–53 in Gore, RD & Garey, J. (eds.) (2010).

Miklowitz, DJ. (2010) *The Bipolar Disorder Survival Guide: What You and Your Family Need to Know.* 2nd edition. The Guilford Press, New York.

Mondimore, FM. (2014) *Bipolar Disorder: A Guide for Patients and Families.* 3rd edition. Johns Hopkins University Press, Baltimore.

Norman, M. "A Little Help From My Friend" pages 61–64 in Gore, RD & Garey, J. (eds.) (2010).

Nye, C. "Almost Contagious" pages 109–112 in Gore, RD & Garey, J. (eds.) (2010).

O'Neal, D. "Why I Write" pages 143–145 in Gore, RD & Garey, J. (eds.) (2010).

Pilkington, A. "Pushing Forward" pages 169–172 in Gore, RD & Garey, J. (eds.) (2010).

Popov, LK. (2004) *A Pace of Grace.* Plume, New York.

Presley, K. "Dealing with Alternative Cloud Patterns" pages 131–134 in Gore, RD & Garey, J. (eds.) (2010).

Price, SE. (2014) *Bipolar Disorder Survival Guide: How to manage your bipolar symptoms, become stable and get your life back.* Sara Elliott Price (self-published).

Richards, P. "You Know Me" pages 135–137 in Gore, RD & Garey, J. (eds.) (2010).

Rowe, NB. "One Sparkling Facet" pages 21–26 in Gore, RD & Garey, J. (eds.) (2010).

Rusczyk, L. "Saturday" pages 11–15 in Gore, RD & Garey, J. (eds.) (2010).

Schaffer, A., Cairney, J., Cheung, A., Veldhuizen, S. & Levitt, A. "Community Survey of Bipolar Disorder in Canada: Lifetime Prevalence and Illness Characteristics" *Canadian Journal of Psychiatry*, Vol. 51, No. 1, January 2006:9–16.

Stearn, S. "Let the Music Be Your Master" pages 155–159 in Gore, RD & Garey, J. (eds.) (2010).

Trudeau, M. (2010) *Changing my mind.* HarperCollins Publishers Ltd., Toronto.

Whetsell, JP. "What They See Is What You Get: On the (Mis)Diagnosis, Un-Diagnosis, and Re-Diagnosis of Bipolar Disorder" pages 55–59 in Gore, RD & Garey, J. (eds.) (2010).

Weil, J. "Bipolar Disorder: A Mother's Perspective" pages 85–91 in Gore, RD & Garey, J. (eds.) (2010).

Williams, M., Teasdale, J., Segal, Z. & Kabat-Zinn, J. (2007) *The mindful way through depression: Freeing yourself from chronic unhappiness.* The Guilford Press, New York.

Yorkey, B. (2010) *Next to Normal.* Theatre Communications Group, New York.

About the author

I was born in South Africa, where I studied nursing and midwifery, then sociology, and finally got a doctorate in public health and adult education. I also got post-graduate qualifications in nursing administration, nursing education and community health. I worked in the Department of Community Health at the University of the Witwatersrand in Johannesburg, and during this time, co-edited a series of three public health textbooks published by Oxford University Press, and numerous scholarly articles about medical education, primary health care, and other topics.

My husband, Rob Collins and I moved to Canada in 1988 and we co-authored *Self-directed learning: critical practice*, published by Kogan Page in London (UK) in 1989. In 1993, Rob and I co-authored another book, *One World, One Earth: Educating Children for Social Responsibility*, published by New Society Publishers, Canada. During these early years in Canada, I was an at-home mother to 3 young children and two teenaged stepchildren. In 1995 I published another book, *Pesticide Bylaws: why we need them; how to get them*, partially funded by the Quebec government. In the mid 1990s, I started working outside the home again, and focused on public health consulting work. Rob and I both work mainly with Indigenous communities, mostly Inuit communities in the far north, and various First Nations communities. We've co-authored numerous resources about issues of public health concern to Indigenous communities, especially tobacco reduction.

After over 13 years of a very active career managing numerous health projects and travelling to all corners of the

Canadian Arctic, in 2008 I was struck with bipolar disorder at age 51. In *Mad Like Me: Travels in Bipolar Country* I aim to bring readers along with me for the wild ride through bipolar country. By retelling events with unblinking honesty, I hope to demystify this greatly misunderstood mental illness, and humanize the people it affects. The stigma against mental illness of all kinds in all ages must end!

For videos, photos and media links about me, my family and the book, please visit merrylhammond.com.

Please review!

Thanks so much for reading this!

As I said at the start, we're actively seeking reviews both for my website – merrylhammond.com (which includes video clips, links to radio and media interviews, etc.) – and for Amazon. (You're only eligible to post reviews if you have an active Amazon account.) If you're not familiar with posting reviews on Amazon, it's really easy:

1. Please google Amazon, choose "Kindle Store" in the drop-down menu at the top left of the page and type *Mad Like Me* in the search bar.

2. Click on the cover or the title of *Mad Like Me: Travels in Bipolar Country*. This will open the book's "detail page" with prices, product details, etc.

3. Scroll down past all the ads until you see the heading "Customer reviews" with 5 yellow stars below it. Just to the right of those stars is a small white box that says "Write a customer review". Click that box, and you'll be asked to sign in to your Amazon account.

4. Now you're ready to post a review. Write a sentence or two that will convey your main feelings about the book; draft a brief headline for your review; and give it a star rating (from one to five where 5 is excellent). That's it!

Every additional review really helps. So please help spread the word about stigma reduction if you feel this book is worth sharing. Join the movement!

Thanks very much!

Merryl Hammond

CPSIA information can be obtained
at www.ICGtesting.com
Printed in the USA
LVHW041011040819
626455LV00017B/892